Wiley
Nursing
Concept
Modules

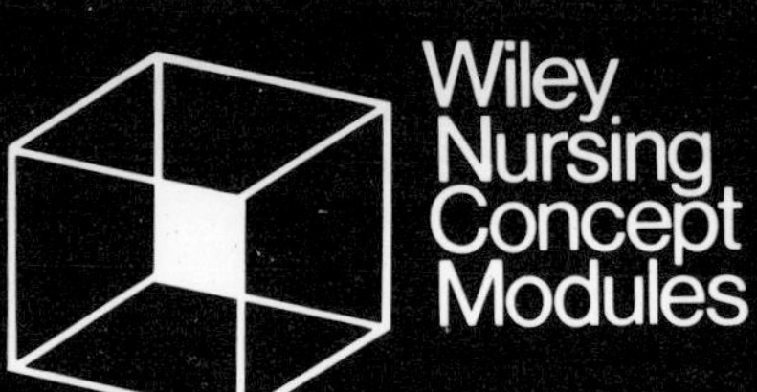

Nutrition in Nursing

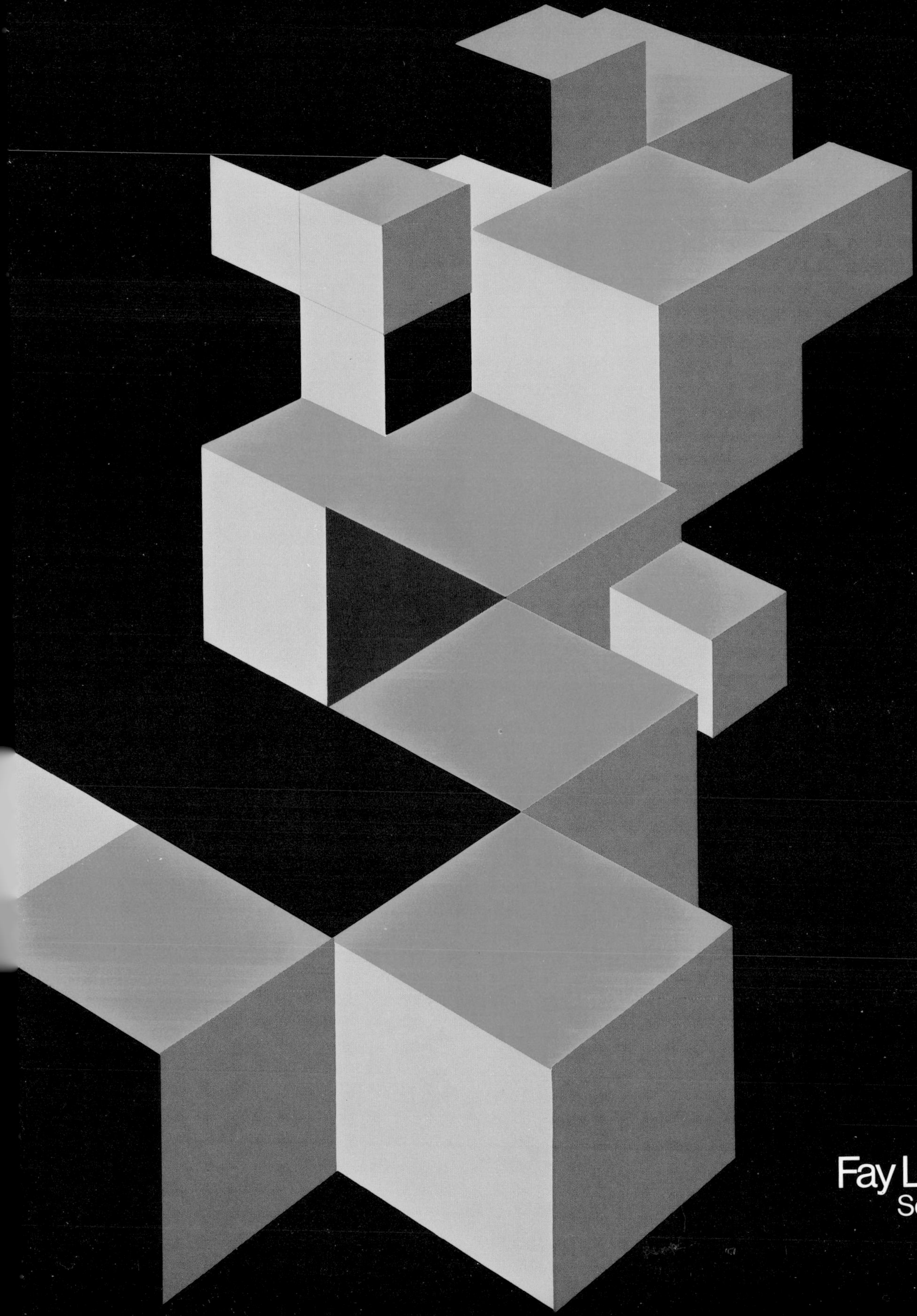

Fay L. Bower
Series Editor

Nutrition in Nursing

tm

Nutrition in Nursing

Series Editor and Consultant:

FAY L. BOWER, R.N., M.S.N.

Chairperson
School of Nursing
San Jose State University
San Jose, California

Wiley Nursing Concept Module

A Wiley Medical Publication

John Wiley & Sons

New York/Chichester
Brisbane/Toronto

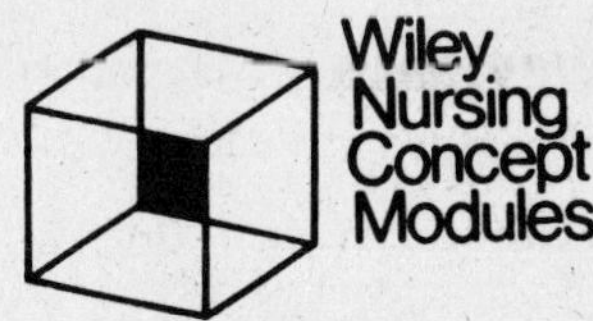

Library of Congress Cataloging in Publication Data:

Main entry under title:

Nutrition in nursing.

(Wiley nursing concept module)
1. Nutrition. 2. Malnutrition. 3. Food consumption. 4. Diet therapy. 5. Reducing diets. 6. Nursing. I. Bower, Fay Louise. II. Series: Wiley nursing concept modules. [DNLM: 1. Nutrition--Nursing texts. 2. Nutrition disorders--Nursing texts. QU145.3 N9763]

RA784.N846 612'.3 79-10562
ISBN 0-471-04124-6

Printed in the United States of America

10 9 8 7 6 5 4 3 2 1

CONTRIBUTORS

JULIE M. MILNE, M.S., R.D.
Nutrition and Diet Therapy Instructor
Wesley-Passavant School of Nursing
Northwestern Memorial Hospital
Chicago, Illinois

PEGGY STANFIELD, M.S., R.D.
Associate Professor
Department of Nursing
College of Southern Idaho
Twin Falls, Idaho

SERIES PREFACE

During the last decade there have been major changes in instructional formats. In an attempt to provide learning experiences that meet individual needs and abilities, educators have tried various instructional methods such as audiotutorial learning, independent study, and most recently, learning modules. Students of all ages, studying a wide variety of subjects, have been introduced to modular programs.

Of all the new instructional approaches, learning modules have taken the lead. Administrators and teachers feel encouraged about them because they permit the implementation of learning principles. Their popularity is also partly due to their flexibility for learner use and their economic use of teacher time. Teachers employing modules can spend time with the slower learners while the faster learners proceed on their own.

The term *module* did not originate in the field of education. The term has various meanings--components of television sets, parts of a spacecraft, construction units of a building. In education *module* refers to a self-contained package dealing with a single conceptual entity that can be completed at a time and place determined by the learner.

This volume is a collection of learning modules about a specific subject. Each module in the book deals with a portion of the subject and follows the same format: pretest, learning objectives, directions, activities, progress checks, and posttest. The modules are designed for independent learner use, but they can also be used as a basis for seminars. Some of the learning modules refer the learner to media-tapes, films, slides, books, or games. All the modules suggest learning activities.

This volume of modules can be used in schools of nursing by students and teachers and by nurses in staff development programs. They were designed to fit into any curriculum pattern and any staff development program.

Praise and thanks are due the authors of the modules, who have prepared them from expert knowledge of the contents and from a desire to make learning enjoyable and rewarding. Special thanks to the many students, too many to list here, who have encouraged me to publish modules for their use. Their suggestions, critiques, and encouragement have made this book a reality.

Fay L. Bower

MODULES

Nutrition Today: An Overview

JULIE M. MILNE, M.S., R.D.

Contents

INTRODUCTION

Nutrition has been recognized as one of man's basic needs since the days of Florence Nightingale. She felt that it was the physician's place to prescribe the food for the patient, but that the art and science of feeding the ill was an essential part of nursing care.[1] The role of the nurse and the knowledge base about nutrition have changed drastically since the 1850's and will no doubt continue to do so. Nurses of today do more than carry out the orders of physicians. They are becoming more involved in education, not only for the patient, but also for the consumer; in collaborating with professional colleagues in the planning and delivery of total health care needs; and in diagnostic work. With this greater independence and responsibility comes a need for deeper understanding of nutrition's influence upon the physiological status of man.

One cannot open a women's magazine or a newspaper without being aware of the increased public interest and concern about nutrition--how it will affect health, cure ills, and so on. Although nutrition is not a cause of, nor a cure-all for, all medical disorders, we as health professionals need to be aware of the role that good nutrition plays in maintaining man's biopsychosocial health.

The following activities have been designed to help the reader become more aware of present dietary trends in the United States, of their health implications, and of possible nursing interventions.

PREREQUISITES FOR THIS MODULE

Chapters on dietary guides, proteins, carbohydrates, lipids, and energy metabolism from one of the texts listed in the References will increase your understanding of this module. You will be

---

[1]Cooper, L., "Florence Nightingale's Contribution to Dietetics," *Journal of American Dietetics*, A, 121, 1954.

responsible for applying knowledge from these areas in the Activities and Progress Checks.

TERMINAL OBJECTIVES

Upon the completion of this module, the learner will be able to

1. Define the term *nutrition*.
2. Assess the nutritive value of selected foods.
3. Identify dietary trends in the United States during the past four decades that have affected our patterns of living.
4. Relate present dietary trends to health implications.
5. Identify suggestions made by the Senate Select Committee on Human Needs to meet recommended dietary goals.
6. Recognize the nurse's nutrition interventions in primary, secondary, and tertiary health care.
7. Identify agencies that have reliable nutrition information available for the consumer.

PRETEST

Please complete the following pretest. If you can correctly answer 80% of the questions, you may proceed to the next module, as you will have demonstrated knowledge of this module. If you cannot correctly answer at least 80% of the questions, proceed to page 12.

1. Define *nutrition*.

2. Listed below are items in four grocery carts:

Cart 1

Baking potatoes
Eggs
Half and half (cream)
Iceberg lettuce
Sirloin steak
Whole milk

Cart 2

Cabbage
Cornbread
Green beans
Low-fat yogurt
Pinto beans
Tomatoes

Cart 3

Cheddar cheese
Cornflakes
Macaroni
Margarine
Skim milk
Tunafish

Cart 4

Chicken livers
Cottage cheese
Dried apricots
Instant mashed potatoes
Peanut butter
Sweet potatoes

Which of these carts contains *at least one food* from each of the Basic Four Food Groups? Circle the correct answer.

a) 1
b) 2
c) 3
d) 4

3. Which of the carts in question 2 would be *MOST hazardous* to a person eating a low-fat, low-cholesterol diet?

   a) 1
   b) 2
   c) 3
   d) 4

4. In terms of the daily requirement for the fruit and vegetable group of the Basic Four, a healthy 65-year-old man, in comparison with a healthy adolescent male, will need

   a) One less serving of a fruit.
   b) One less serving of a vegetable.
   c) One less serving of both fruit and vegetable.
   d) The same number of servings of fruit and vegetable.

5. A fast-food operation serves the following items:

   Special Burger (4 oz fried ground beef patty, mayonnaise, catsup, mustard, pickle on a poppyseed bun)

   Cheeseburger (2 oz fried ground beef patty with 1 oz American cheese on a hamburger bun)

   Hamburger (2 oz fried ground beef patty on a hamburger bun)

   Fish Filet (4 oz fried white fish filet, tartar sauce, coleslaw, on a poppyseed bun)

   French Fries

   Milkshakes: Chocolate, Strawberry, Vanilla

   Milk: Whole, Chocolate

Coke, Sprite, Orange, Root Beer

Coffee, Tea

Fried Pies: Apple, Cherry

Evaluate these foods as a group by listing their nutritional advantages and/or disadvantages.

Advantages	Disadvantages

6. Which of the following organizations would provide the *most* reliable information for the consumer and why?

    a) The American Dietetic Association

    b) American Meat Institute

    c) Cereal Institute, Inc.

    d) Food and Drug Administration

    e) General Mills, Consumer Center

    f) U.S. Department of Agriculture

Why?

7. Dietary trends in the United States have been influenced by changes in our style of living. Which of the following social developments might affect our style of living?

   1) Families eating more meals at home

   2) Mass media advertising

   3) More leisure time due to working fewer hours

   4) People moving from urban to rural communities

   Circle the correct answer.

   a) 1 and 2 c) 2 and 4

   b) 2 and 3 d) 3 and 4

Match the dietary trends listed below with possible health implications. There may be more than one answer per dietary trend.

<u>Health Implications</u>

a) Weight loss

b) Weight gain, obesity

c) Increased serum fats, cholesterol, lipoproteins

d) Increased polyunsaturated fats

e) Chronic constipation

f) Cancer of the colon

g) Coronary heart disease

h) Hypertension

i) Dental caries

Dietary Trends

8. _____ Caloric intake the same, energy expenditure less

9. _____ Increased consumption of animal versus plant protein

10. _____ Reduced consumption of starches, flour and cereals, fiber

11. _____ Increased consumption of all fats

12. _____ Increased consumption of refined sugars

13. Which of the following suggestions were made by the Senate Select Committee on Human Needs to meet their recommended dietary goals?

    1) Decrease consumption of salt and foods high in salt.

    2) Decrease consumption of foods high in refined and other processed sugars.

    3) Except for young children, substitute lowfat and skim milk for whole milk.

    4) Substitute saturated fats for polyunsaturated fats.

    5) Increase intake of red meats and decrease intake of poultry and fish.

    6) Decrease intake of fruits, vegetables, and whole grains.

    Circle the correct answer.

    a) 2, 3, and 6 c) 2, 3, and 4

    b) 3, 4, and 5 d) 1, 2, and 3

Match the following nursing interventions with the level of preventive health care.

Levels of Preventive Health Care

a) Primary

b) Secondary

c) Tertiary

Nursing Interventions

14. _____ Be certain iron sulfate is ordered for a patient with low hemoglobin and hematocrit levels.

15. _____ Assist a client in making arrangements to receive food stamps.

16. _____ Secure nipple for feeding an infant with a cleft palate.

17. _____ Teach mothers in a prenatal clinic how to bathe a baby.

18. _____ Assist a new diabetic in learning how to administer insulin.

19. _____ Teach a newly diagnosed cardiac patient about menu planning for a low sodium content.

ANSWERS

1. *Nutrition.* Nutrition is "the science of foods, the nutrients and other substances therein; their action, interaction, and balance in relationship to health and disease; the processes by which the organism ingests, digests, absorbs, transports, and utilizes nutrients and disposes

of their end products. In addition, nutrition must be concerned with social, economic, cultural, and psychological implications of food and eating."

2. b

3. a

4. d

5. Advantages:

    Good protein
    Serves milk

   Disadvantages:

    High in calories
    High in saturated fat
    Low in vitamins A and C
    Low in fiber and roughage
    We don't know exactly what products or additives are in the meat patties, milkshakes, and so on that could cause problems for the consumer with allergies or a metabolic abnormality.

6. a, d, and f
   The other three are industry related. Consumer information published by these organizations might be aimed at trying to sell a product and might not speak of the negative health implications of their products.

7. b

8. b

9. c, g, h

10. c, e, f

11. c, g

12. c, i

13. d

14. b

15. a

16. c

17. a

18. b

19. a

ACTIVITY 1
UNITED STATES DIETARY TRENDS

If one were to ask a nonmedical person what the word *nutrition* means, the answer would probably be, "It's the food I eat." Webster defines nutrition as "the act or process of nourishing or being nourished,"[2] a very nonspecific definition. How does man nourish himself? What does he consider good nourishment? In the 1960's, nutritionists from the United States Department of Agriculture (U.S.D.A.) developed "The Daily Food Guide"[3] (Basic Four Food Groups) and it has been updated by the National Dairy Council (see Table 1) to give Americans some guidelines for meeting their daily nutritional requirements. Do people follow the Basic Four Food Groups in planning what they eat?

TABLE 1

GUIDE TO GOOD EATING: A Recommended Daily Pattern[4]

Milk Group

Children	3 or more cups
Teenagers	4 or more cups
Adults	2 or more cups
Pregnant women	4 or more cups
Lactating women	4 or more cups

Calcium equivalents for 1 cup milk include:

1 cup yogurt
1½ oz cheddar cheese
1 cup pudding
1 3/4 cups ice cream
2 cups cottage cheese

---

[2]*Webster's Third New International Dictionary* (Springfield, Mass.: G. & C. Merriam Company, 1961.

[3]*Consumer and Food Economics Research Division Agriculture Research Service*, rev. ed. (Washington, D.C.: 1964).

[4]Modified from publication B164 of the National Dairy Council, Rosemont, Ill., 1977.

TABLE 1 (continued)

Meat Group

Two or more 2 oz servings cooked, lean meat. During pregnancy, three 2 oz servings are recommended.

Beef, veal, pork, lamb, poultry, fish.

As alternates--eggs, cheese, dried beans, peas, peanut butter, soy extenders, nuts.

Vegetable-Fruit Group

Four or more servings.

A citrus fruit is recommended daily for vitamin C. A dark green leafy, or orange vegetable or fruit is recommended three or four times weekly for vitamin A.

Bread-Cereal Group

Four or more servings whole grain, enriched, or fortified.

Ready-to-eat and cooked cereals, pasta, crackers, grits, rice.

Other Group

To round out meals and meet energy needs, most everyone will use some foods not specified in the Basic Four Food Groups. Such foods include bakery products that are not whole grain or enriched; sugars; butter, margarine, and other fats; alcoholic beverages; many processed snack foods; and so on. Amounts of foods eaten in this group should be determined by individual caloric needs. The recommended servings from the Basic Four Food Groups for adults supply about 1200 Calories.

Over the past ten to fifteen years, several epidemiological and food-disappearance studies have been conducted to determine what people in the United States are eating. Data from these studies, the Survey of Preschool Children,[5] the Ten State

---

[5]Owen, G.M., et al., "A study of nutritional status of preschool children in the United States, 1968-70," *Pediatrics*, 53: 597.

Nutrition Survey,[6] the HANES Survey,[7] and the Compendium of Nutritional Status Surveys[8] all tend to confirm that as a nation, Americans are consuming more than the Basic Four Food Groups suggest. The following changes have been noted in American eating habits over the past four decades.

1. Calorie consumption has remained essentially the same, although energy expenditure has declined as our society has become more mechanized. This has resulted in weight increase.

2. A mechanized, urban society has made America more affluent, giving people more money to spend on food, especially protein. Surprisingly, the proportion of Calories obtained from protein today is similar to that in 1910, about 10 percent. However, there has been a shift in the type of protein consumed. Today a higher proportion is consumed from animal sources--meat, poultry, fish, eggs, and dairy products--and a smaller proportion is derived from grain and other vegetable sources. Many economists would like to see Americans consume more vegetable proteins again, as we would be "reaping" greater utilization and efficiency from our farm lands.

3. The American population as a whole is also consuming more than 40 percent of their Calories as fat. This figure has been steadily increasing over the past 40 years. The National Restaurant Association estimates that in our mobile, working society, Americans eat more than half of their meals away from home. Analyze menus from fast-food operations and restaurants. What

---

[6]Department of Health, Education and Welfare, *Ten State Nutrition Survey, 1968-70*, Publication No. (HMS) 72-8130, 72-8131.

[7]Abraham, S., et al., *Preliminary Findings of the First Health and Nutrition Examination Survey, United States, 1971-72*, Dietary Intake and Biochemical Findings Publication No. (HRA) 74-1219-1 (Washington, D.C.: Department of Health, Education and Welfare, 1974).

[8]Kelsay, J.L., *A Compendium of Nutritional Status Studies and Dietary Evaluation Studies Conducted in the U.S., 1957-67*.

percentage of plain broiled or baked foods do you see, as opposed to those with fancy sauces or gravies on top? The restaurant syndrome has had a tremendous influence on fat consumption. Also, with the increase in the consumption of animal proteins, the cholesterol levels have risen slightly. With increased use of vegetable oils, there has been a more noticeable increase in polyunsaturated fats, especially over the past 20 years.

4. There has been a decline in carbohydrate consumption during the past four decades together with a shift in the types of carbohydrates consumed. The first major alteration is a marked decline in the consumption of starches--that is, flour and cereal grain products--accompanied by a decrease in fiber intake. Second, as one might suspect after taking a look at Saturday morning television commercials, magazine advertisements and coupons, or the contents sold in most vending machines, there has been a rise in total and refined sugar consumption, including alcohol.

5. Thanks in part to the government enrichment programs (in the 1940's, the addition of iron, riboflavin, niacin, and thiamin to processed flours and cereals and of vitamin A to margarine; in the 1930's, the fortifying of milk with Vitamin D; and the earlier addition of iodine to salt), the consumption of many of the vitamins and minerals has increased over the past century.

What effect, if any, do you think these changes in the American diet have had on our health? This will be discussed in Activity 2. But first, check your progress on Activity 1.

PROGRESS CHECK

1. Using an authoritative resource, construct a scientific definition for *nutrition*.

2. If American Calorie consumption remains the same and energy intake decreases, which of the following will occur?

   a) Weight will remain the same.

   b) Weight will increase.

   c) Weight will decrease.

3. A shift in protein consumption from vegetable to animal protein has resulted in which of the following?

   1) Better utilization of our agricultural land.

   2) Intake of fewer Calories.

   3) More money out of the consumer's pocket for protein.

   4) A higher intake of saturated fats and cholesterol.

   Circle the correct answer.

   a) 1 and 2

   b) 3 and 4

   c) 2, 3, and 4

   d) All of the above

4. List some of the physiological dangers of the increased consumption of refined sugars in the American diet.

5. M.M., a 35-year-old housewife, 5 ft 3 in, 125 lb, tells you that her average food intake for one day includes the following:

   Breakfast: Fried eggs, 2
   Bacon, 2 strips
   Sweetroll with butter
   Coffee with cream

   Lunch: Ham salad sandwich on rye bread with mayonnaise
   Potato chips
   Brownie
   Cola beverage

   Dinner: Fried chicken
   Mashed potatoes with gravy
   Peas and mushrooms in butter sauce
   Gelatin salad with bananas
   Apple pie with a scoop of vanilla ice cream
   Hot tea with sugar

   Before bed: Apple pie, 1 slice

   a) Evaluate the diet according to the Basic Four Food Groups. Were all requirements met?

b) Which dietary trends discussed in this activity do you see being exhibited in M.M.'s diet?

c) Modify M.M.'s diet to meet the Basic Four Food Groups.

d) Outline a teaching plan for M.M. that would alleviate some of the nutrition problems posed by her present diet.

6. *Increase your consumer awareness.* Watch Saturday morning children's television programs, including the advertising. Read food advertisements, including coupons, in magazines and newspapers. Check what is sold in your school, hospital, or business vending machines.

   a) What types of foods are advertised?

   b) How many of the foods promoted are junk foods --that is, have little nutritional value other than Calories?

   c) What do you think of the psychology behind advertising on television and in magazines?

   d) Do you think there is anything you can do to alter advertising? If so, what?

e) What kinds of food are in the vending machines? If it is mainly junk food, do you think you can do anything about seeing that more nutritional foods are placed in vending machines?

ANSWERS

1. *Nutrition*. Nutrition is "the science of foods, the nutrients and other substances therein; their action, interaction, and balance in relationship to health and disease; the processes by which the organism ingests, digests, absorbs, transports, and utilizes nutrients and disposes of their end products. In addition, nutrition must be concerned with social, economic, cultural, and psychological implications of food and eating."

2. b

3. b

4. Consumption of refined sugars can lead to dental caries if the person does not practice excellent oral hygiene.

   Use of refined sugars can lead to an increased incidence of diabetes.

   For some of the population, an intake of refined sugars can lead to an increase in levels of lipoproteins (cholesterol and triglycerides).

5. a) Milk--needs at least 1½ more cups; is getting milk only in ice cream.

   Meat--adequate; eggs, ham, chicken.

   Vegetable and Fruit--four servings (mashed potatoes, peas and mushrooms, banana, apple in pie). While potatoes that are not overly cooked are a good source of vitamin C, no excellent source of vitamin C, such as a citrus fruit, was consumed. An excellent source of vitamin A is also needed.

   Bread and Cereal--needs one more serving; consumed two slices of rye bread and one sweet roll. While the sweet roll is enriched, it does have a high content of refined sugars, and some nutritionists might prefer to place it in the "Other" group.

   Other (mainly Calories without other nutritional value)--potato chips, brownie, pie crust, gelatin; bacon, cream, butter, gravy, mayonnaise, butter sauce; sugar cola beverage; coffee; tea.

   b) Increased intake of animal protein: eggs, ham salad, chicken.

   Increased intake of fat: bacon, butter (sauce), cream, mayonnaise; fat incorporated in potato chips, brownie, fried chicken, gravy, pie, and ice cream.

Decreased intake of starches, fiber: does not meet Basic Four requirements in Bread-Cereal Group; the only whole grain product is rye bread; no fresh fruits or vegetables

Increased intake of refined sugars: sweet roll, brownie, cola, gelatin salad, apple pie, table sugar.

c) Breakfast: ½ fresh grapefruit
1 poached egg on 1 slice whole wheat toast with 1 tsp vegetable-oil margarine
Coffee with skim milk
1 cup skim milk

Lunch: Tuna salad sandwich on 2 slices rye bread with lettuce and tomato
Raw celery and carrot sticks, radishes
Golden delicious apple
1 cup skim milk

Dinner: Baked chicken
Baked sweet potatoes with 1 tsp vegetable-oil margarine
Peas and mushrooms seasoned with dillweed
Tossed salad with oil and vinegar dressing
Low-fat yogurt blended with fresh strawberries
Hot tea with lemon

d) Suggest to M.M. that she

(1) Reduce her intake from the "Other" group; that is, reduce the amounts of fats (cream, bacon, butter, mayonnaise, gravy), refined sugars (brownies, pie), and empty-Calorie foods (cola).

(2) Become familiar with her spice shelf and use spices, which have no Calories, instead of high-Calorie fats to flavor meats and vegetables.

(3) Bake, broil, roast, or stew meats. Do not fry or serve with gravies or sauces.

(4) Substitute whole grain or enriched bread/cereal products for sugary starches such as donuts, sweet rolls, and coffeecakes.

(5) Use fresh fruit or plain yogurt mixed with fresh fruit instead of high-Calorie desserts.

(6) Eat crisp, fresh vegetables instead of crisp junk food such as potato chips or corn chips.

(7) Eat fresh fruit or fruit packed in water or its own juice rather than fruit packed in syrups.

6. d) What can you do about altering some of the advertising pertaining to foods?

You can work for the regulation of television advertising of sugared snacks aimed at children. You, personally or with your professional organization, could join the campaign being carried on by many health professionals --such as the Center for Science in Public Interest, the members of the Society for Nutrition Education, and Action for Children's Television--who have petitioned the Federal Trade Commission to ban advertising of sugared snacks and candy on children's programming.

You and your group could also boycott the sale of sugared snacks, candy, desserts, and the like, whether advertised on television or in a magazine or newspaper. Such advertising includes coupons that offer a monetary discount when you purchase any of these items.

e) Placement of nutritious foods in vending machines:

Again, you could boycott machines that contain junk foods. You could also ask those who have control over the vending machines to remove the junk foods and put in machines that contain more nutritious foods such as milk, juices, and sandwiches. Many parents all across the nation have petitioned their respective school boards to remove all vending machines from the school unless they vend nutritious foods such as milk, juice, apples, and oranges.

As a nurse and health professional, be aware that your community will be looking up to you for advice and will hold your medical opinion in high regard. Helping to promote a cause such as the placement of nutritious foods in school vending machines can be just as important in promoting health as participating in a polio vaccination campaign.

Activity 2

HEALTH IMPLICATIONS OF CHANGING FOOD PATTERNS

Many health professionals believe that changes in eating patterns over the past four decades have greatly contributed to major health problems in the United States today.

Obesity. It is estimated that one out of two Americans is overweight. Though calorie consumption has remained essentially the same over the past four decades, the decline in energy expenditure has led to obesity.

Coronary health disease and hypertension. These conditions have been related to a diet high in animal protein, which is naturally accompanied by an increased intake of saturated fats, cholesterol, and sodium. Some studies also suggest that the reduced consumption of fiber has played a role in the increase of serum cholesterol. And for some of the population, an increased intake of refined sugar may lead to an increase in lipoproteins.

Cancer. The relationship between cancer and diet is being studied, but research is still in very early stages, as most of the investigations done thus far have been epidemiological. Among the relationships being studied are those of dietary fiber to cancer of the colon as well as diverticulitis and chronic constipation, and of cholesterol to cancer of the breast.

Diabetes. It has been suggested that diabetes may be related to an increased consumption of refined sugars together with decreased energy expenditure, leading to obesity.

Dental caries. Caries have been definitely linked to an increased intake of refined sugars, when not accompanied by excellent oral hygiene.

These aspects of nutrition came into the limelight in February, 1977, when the Senate Select Committee on Nutrition and Human Needs recommended that the United States adopt and institute national nutrition goals that would maintain health and prevent disease.[9] The goals suggested by the Committee were studied by numerous individuals and associations in the health professions. Based upon their criticisms, suggestions, and research, the goals were revised as stated below and presented to the public in December, 1977.[10]

1. To avoid obesity, consume only as much energy (calories) as is expended; if overweight, decrease energy intake and increase energy expenditure.

2. Increase the consumption of complex carbohydrates and "naturally occurring" sugars from

[9]Select Committee on Nutrition and Human Needs, U.S. Senate, *Dietary Goals for the United States*, February 1977.

[10]Select Committee on Nutrition and Human Needs, U.S. Senate, *Dietary Goals for the United States*, 2nd ed., December 1977.

about 28% of energy intake to about 48% of energy intake.

3. Reduce the consumption of refined and processed sugars by about 45% to account for about 10% of total energy intake.

4. Reduce overall fat consumption from about 40% to about 30% of energy intake.

5. Reduce saturated fat consumption to account for about 10% of total energy intake; and balance that with polyunsaturated and monounsaturated fats, which should account for about 10% of energy intake each.

6. Reduce cholesterol consumption to about 300 mg a day.

7. Limit the intake of sodium by reducing the intake of salt to about 5 g a day.

In order to achieve these goals, the Committee suggested the following changes in food selection and preparation:

1. Increase consumption of fruits and vegetables and whole grains.

2. Decrease consumption of refined and other processed sugars and foods high in such sugars.

3. Decrease consumption of foods high in total fat and partially replace saturated fats, whether obtained from animal or vegetable sources, with polyunsaturated fats.

4. Decrease consumption of animal fat and choose meats, poultry, and fish that will reduce saturated fat intake.

5. Except for young children, substitute low-fat and nonfat milk for whole milk and low-fat dairy products for high-fat dairy products.

6. Decrease consumption of butterfat, eggs, and other high-cholesterol sources. Some

consideration should be given to easing the cholesterol goal for premenopausal women, young children, and the elderly in order to obtain the nutritional benefits of eggs in the diet.

7. Decrease consumption of salt and foods high in salt content.

These goals will not *guarantee* complete protection from the major killer diseases discussed earlier; however, they will increase the *probability* of improved protection.

To assist the population in meeting these dietary goals, the Committee made recommendations for action by Congress:[11]

1. Provide money for a public education program in nutrition based on the listed (or similar) dietary goals, with an initial minimum period of five years for promoting them.

The need for nutrition education has been recognized in other federal programs, such as the Food Stamp Program and the Special Supplemental Food Program for Women, Infants and Children (WIC). Studies conducted in various WIC programs have proven that merely providing food to help the recipients meet their special nutritional needs was not in itself sufficient; education was also needed to help them learn wise family eating habits. In 1976, WIC was the first federally funded feeding program to receive monies for nutrition education.

Some health professionals are also trying to get a bill through Congress that would institute nutrition education programs in schools (kindergarten through grade 12), with the programs in each community being headed by a nutrition education specialist. The U.S. Department of Agriculture made $26 million available during the 1978 fiscal year to states to conduct a new

---

[11]"Senate Committee Lists Dietary Goals for U.S.," *Journal of the American Dietetic Association*, 70: 449 (1977).

nutrition education and training program. Considering the unfavorable eating patterns and health implications mentioned previously, one can readily see the importance of sound nutrition education early in childhood, before too many bad eating habits are established.

2. Require labeling for *all* foods, with information on percent and type of fats, percent of sugar, milligrams of cholesterol and of salt, caloric content, and a complete list of food additives. This would be helpful not only in the prevention of the major diseases listed earlier, but also for people with food allergies.

3. Fund joint studies and pilot projects by the USDA and the Department of Health, Education and Welfare (DHEW) to develop new techniques in food processing and institutional and home meal preparation aimed at reducing risk factors in the diet.

   Presently there is a good deal of sodium and sometimes hidden fat in convenience/processed foods. Think of all the canned fruits packed in heavy syrups, too. And one never really knows for sure what is in institutional food.

4. Increase funding for human nutrition research by the USDA and establish a committee to coordinate such research undertaken by the USDA and the DHEW.

All of this may look beautiful on paper. Adhering to these Dietary Goals certainly shouldn't be physiologically dangerous to anyone. Yet, many health professionals are questioning the Dietary Goals as they are set forth. As a result, the goals have not been passed by Congress.

In a newsletter to its members, the Board of Directors of the Society for Nutrition Education stated its concern "that the evidence cited in the Dietary Goals document is largely limited to epidemiological data and food disappearance studies (those studies listed in Activity 1) which result in population needs rather than individual goals."[12] This statement was also in agreement with the American Medical Association's position that the evidence is not conclusive.[13] In other words, epidemiological research investigates populations. There are no control groups, so there could be a million and one variables affecting what is being investigated--in this case the relationship of diet to specific diseases. Therefore, it is not scientifically or statistically valid to relate some of the nutritional practices to specific disease states until more controlled research is completed.

The importance of national dietary goals should not be overshadowed by this discussion of the appropriateness of the data used in determining the goals. This attempt by the federal government to develop a primary prevention program for health care has hopefully alerted all health professionals to the importance of good nutrition in the prevention of certain diseases.

However, this point about the research should remind us to critique carefully everything that we read, whether in a women's magazine, a newspaper, or a professional journal. Remember to look at the author's credentials, the methodology of the study conducted, and the validity of the statistics.

In Activity 3, the nurse's role in preventive health care will be explored. First, check your progress on Activity 2.

PROGRESS CHECK

1. Why do some health professionals *not* consider information obtained from epidemiological studies as reliable?

---

[12]Society for Nutrition Education, Board of Directors, "Statement on the Dietary Goals for the U.S.," *SNE Communicator*, 8: 6, June 1977.

[13]American Medical Association, "Statement to the Select Committee on Nutrition and Human Needs," U.S. Senate, April 18, 1977.

Correlate the possible health implications listed below with the dietary trends that follow.

Health Implications

a) Weight loss

b) Weight gain, obesity

c) Increased serum fats, cholesterol, lipoproteins

d) Increased polyunsaturated fats

e) Chronic constipation

f) Cancer of the colon

g) Coronary heart disease

h) Hypertension

i) Dental caries

Dietary Trends

2. _____ Caloric intake the same, energy expenditure less

3. _____ Increased consumption of animal versus plant protein

4. _____ Reduced consumption of starches, flour and cereals, fiber

5. _____ Increased consumption of all fats, including cholesterol

6. _____ Increased consumption of refined sugars

ANSWERS

1. There are no controls, and so one can never be certain of which variables affect the relationships.

2. b

3. c, g, h

4. c, e, f

5. c, g

6. c, i

ACTIVITY 3
NURSING INTERVENTIONS: PRIMARY, SECONDARY, TERTIARY

Thus far in this module, we have considered American dietary patterns and their possible health implications. The reader should have gathered that Americans are not eating what is physiologically best for them, and health care providers and the government are greatly concerned with educating the public to alter their eating habits in order to prevent the occurrence of the nation's major diseases. In other words, preventive health care needs to encompass nutrition.

Preventive health care takes place on three levels: primary, secondary, and tertiary. The objectives of the three levels are

1. *Primary prevention*
   a. Averts the occurrence of disease.
   b. Protects the general health and well-being of individuals with specific health measures.
2. *Secondary prevention*
   a. Utilizes early diagnosis to prevent further complications and disabilities.
   b. Provides prompt treatment to arrest the disease process.

3. *Tertiary prevention*
    a. Provides facilities for retraining and education for the maximum use of the patient's remaining capacities.
    b. Educates the public and industry to utilize rehabilitated persons.[14]

The first two activities in this module discussed several government primary prevention nutrition programs that have been developed to avert the occurrence of diseases of malnutrition. These programs, which include food enrichment programs and the Food Stamp and WIC programs, are often called "equalization" programs, as they attempt to provide food to and increase the nutritional status of people on low or limited incomes at a lower price than those people in high income brackets would have to pay. Other nutrition equalization programs are Head Start preschool programs, the Type A school lunch program and breakfast programs, and the Title VII Nutrition Program of the Older Americans Act. Because regulations for these programs change periodically and some vary from one region of the country to another, it would be best for the reader to call the local health department, city hall, or Visiting Nurse Association to find out which of the above programs are operating and what their individual regulations are for eligibility to participate.

AWARENESS on the part of the nurse is vital for *primary prevention*. Today's nurse is a specialist. Although the nurse cannot be expected to be a dietitian, *awareness* of the following points will help alleviate disease and promote the health of every patient.

1. *Working knowledge of basic nutrition*

    The nurse in a hospital setting should check the patient's menu after the patient has filled it out to be certain food selections meet the Basic Four Food Groups requirements. If they don't,

---

[14]Tathwell, S., "Levels of Preventive Health Care," Class Handout, Core I, Wesley-Passavant School of Nursing, Chicago, September 1977.

this would be an excellent point from which to begin some nutrition teaching.

The school nurse might speak to health classes about the dangers of some of the fad diets that are being so widely publicized in the media.

The public health nurse might teach a class in prenatal clinics about the importance of good nutrition during pregnancy for the mother and the fetus.

During National Heart Week in February, the industrial nurse might hold classes on the relationship of high-cholesterol and high-sodium diets to coronary heart disease and hypertension. The nurse might also work with the cafeteria manager in planning low-cholesterol, low-sodium menus for the week.

2. *Knowledge of appropriate community resources and referrals*

In order to give all Americans an equal opportunity to receive good nutrition, the nurse should be aware of any federal, state, or local nutrition programs available in the community. If you should find that there are no adequate programs in your community, become involved as a member of the health-care team in getting programs funded.

Many communities have dietitians employed at their public health departments, in Visiting Nurse Associations, and at hospital outpatient clinics who would be available to conduct nutrition education for a minimal fee.

Some larger communities may have a Dial-A-Dietitian service, sponsored by the local dietetic association or local heart, cancer, kidney, or similar associations, where nutrition information is available. Extension nutritionists at state universities are also very involved in community health education.

3. *Knowledge of legislation that affects the nutritional status of Americans*

   As a professional in health care, you can give your congressman vital input regarding health-related issues to help him vote in the best interest of public health, whether it be to appropriate monies for the WIC program, to adopt the Dietary Goals, or to ban the mass-media advertising of candy and other sugary snacks.

For *secondary prevention* the main two objectives are the prevention of further physiological abnormalities and/or the arresting of the disease process. Nursing interventions pertaining to nutrition here would include:

1. Alerting the medical service or physician to abnormal lab values, weight loss or gain, or drug reactions that might require alterations in the diet or vitamin or mineral supplementation. You will study this subject in more detail in the next module.

2. Being aware of the patient's tolerances to the prescribed therapeutic diet, charting intolerances, and being certain that the diet order is changed if need be.

3. Checking the medical record and/or the patient for verification that the patient and/or family has been instructed about the patient's diet before he is discharged, and that he or they comprehend the diet.

Tertiary prevention is primarily concerned with retraining and education for the maximum use of a person's remaining capacities. In dealing with the nutritional aspects of rehabilitation, the nurse should

1. Be certain the individual is fitted or supplied with any eating utensil that will help him feed himself and consume adequate nutrition. This information can be obtained from physical, occupational, and rehabilitation therapy departments or from companies manufacturing the equipment.

2. Advise any bedridden patients, such as paraplegics and quadriplegics, of possible dietary-related side effects of their immobility such as constipation, renal calculi, and skin breakdown, and explain dietary measures to help prevent or alleviate such symptoms.

3. Advise families of stroke, blind, and similarly handicapped patients of the physical and psychological importance of allowing the patient to feed himself, no matter how messy it may be at first.

PROGRESS CHECK

Situation: M.F., 33 years old, has just delivered her first offspring, a set of twins, a boy and a girl. She is three days postpartum. Because her husband's yearly income is only $6000, she used the services of her local prenatal clinic for the pregnancy and delivery. She is breast-feeding the boy and bottle-feeding the girl, who has a slight cleft palate. Both infants are slightly anemic.

List the nursing interventions you would make pertaining to the family's nutritional status on all three levels of preventive health care.

ANSWER

Primary:

Call the public health department to find out:

1. Is there a WIC program in the area?

2. If there is no WIC program, does the health department provide infant formula and/or baby vitamins at cost or free? (Some formula and vitamin manufacturers participate in these programs as a service to the consumer.)

3. Find out if the family is eligible for food stamps, and the cost.

4. Relate the above findings to M.F. and her husband.

5. Teach M.F. about her increased nutritional needs while breast-feeding. Suggest that she check with her clinic obstetrician about continuing her prenatal vitamins while breast-feeding.

Secondary:

1. Have M.F. ask the clinic pediatrician about either vitamins with iron for the boy, formula with iron for the girl, and/or how soon the infants can start the iron-fortified baby cereals.

2. Explain to M.F. the importance of high-iron foods in her own diet, since she is breast-feeding.

Tertiary:

1. Be certain the parents are supplied with sufficient special bottle nipples and shields for feeding the little girl and that they both understand correct feeding procedures for the cleft palate.

SUMMARY

It is important for the nurse to have a good understanding of basic nutrition in order to evaluate the patient's dietary intake and relate it to possible health implications. Only then will the nurse be able to make appropriate interventions to improve the nutritional and health status of the patient.

POSTTEST

1. The science of foods, nutrients, and other substances therein that is concerned with the social, economic, cultural, and psychological implications of eating is

   a) Health.
   b) Nutrition.
   c) Nutritional care.
   d) Nutritional status.

2. The condition of health of the individual as influenced by the utilization of nutrients is

   a) Malnutrition.
   b) Nutritional care.
   c) Undernutrition.
   d) Nutritional status.

3. When the Basic Four are used as a guide in developing a dietary plan for a healthy person, information will be needed about the person's requirements for

   a) Bulk.
   b) Calories.
   c) Fat.
   d) Vitamins.

4. Evaluate the following menu:

   Breakfast

   ½ c orange juice
   1 poached egg
   1 slice whole wheat toast,
   butter, jelly
   coffee, sugar

   Lunch

   1 oz sliced ham
   1 slice rye bread, mayonnaise,
   mustard
   potato chips
   cupcake
   Coke

   Dinner

   3 oz roast beef
   ½ c mashed potatoes with gravy
   2 dinner rolls, butter
   ½ c canned peaches with
   ½ c cottage cheese
   tea, sugar

For an adult, this menu is

1) Adequate.

2) Lacking one serving of milk.

3) Lacking one serving of meat.

4) Lacking one serving from the fruit and vegetable group.

5) Lacking one serving from the bread and cereal group.

Circle the correct answer.

a) 1 only
b) 2 and 3
c) 2 and 4
d) 3 and 4

5. Dietary patterns in the United States have changed greatly over the years along with our style of living. Which of the following could be included as changes in our style of living affecting dietary patterns?

   1) People have moved from urban to rural communities.

   2) Reduction in working hours has made more leisure time available.

   3) Mass media advertising has greatly increased.

   4) Families eat more meals at home.

   Circle the correct answer.

   a) 1 and 2
   b) 1 and 3
   c) 2 and 3
   d) 3 and 4

Correlate the possible health implications listed below with the dietary trends that follow.

Health Implications

a) Weight loss

b) Weight gain, obesity

c) Increased serum fats, cholesterol, lipoproteins

d) Increased polyunsaturated fats

e) Chronic constipation

f) Cancer of the colon

g) Coronary heart disease

h) Hypertension

i) Dental caries

Dietary Trends

6. _____ Caloric intake the same, energy expenditure less

7. _____ Increased consumption of animal versus plant protein

8. _____ Reduced consumption of starches, flour, cereals, and fiber

9. _____ Increased consumption of all fats, including cholesterol

10. _____ Increased consumption of refined sugars

11. Which of the following suggestions were made by the Senate Select Committee on Human Needs to meet their recommended Dietary Goals?

    1) Increase intake of fruits, vegetables, and whole grains.

2) Increase intake of meat and decrease intake of poultry and fish.

3) Substitute saturated fats for polyunsaturated fats.

4) Substitute skim milk for whole milk.

5) Decrease consumption of foods high in sugar.

6) Increase consumption of sodium.

Circle the correct answer.

a) 1, 4, and 5 c) 3, 4, and 5

b) 2, 3, and 4 d) 4, 5, and 6

Match the level of preventive health care with the following nursing interventions.

Levels of Preventive Health Care

a) Primary

b) Secondary

c) Tertiary

Nursing Interventions

12. _____ Be certain iron sulfate is ordered for a patient with low hemoglobin and hematocrit levels.

13. _____ Assist a client in making arrangements to receive Meals-On-Wheels.

14. _____ Secure a sponge around a spoon with masking tape to fit the weakened grasp of a stroke patient.

15. _____ Teach mothers in a pediatric clinic how to make babyfood at home.

16. _____ Assist a new diabetic in understanding his diabetic diet.

17. _____ Teach new mothers how to sterilize infant formula.

ANSWERS

1. b	7. c, g, h	13. a
2. d	8. c, e, f	14. c
3. b	9. c, g	15. a
4. c	10. c, i	16. b
5. c	11. a	17. a
6. b	12. b	

REFERENCES

Anderson, L., M. Dibble, H. Mitchell, and H. Rynbergen. *Nutrition in Nursing*. Philadelphia: J.B. Lippincott, 1972.

Howard, R., and N. Herbold. *Nutrition in Clinical Care*. New York: McGraw-Hill, Inc., 1978.

Krause, M., and M. Hunscher. *Food, Nutrition and Diet Therapy*, 5th ed. Philadelphia: W.B. Saunders Co., 1972.

Mitchell, H., H. Rynbergen, L. Anderson, and M. Dibble. *Nutrition in Health and Disease*, 16th ed. Philadelphia: J.B. Lippincott, 1976.

Robinson, D.H. *Normal and Therapeutic Nutrition*, 15th ed. New York: Macmillan, 1977.

Williams, S.R. *Nutrition and Diet Therapy*, 3rd ed. St. Louis: The C.V. Mosby Co., 1977.

Wilson, E., K. Fisher, and P. Garcia. *Principles of Nutrition*, 4th ed. New York: John Wiley & Sons, 1979.

Malnutrition

JULIE M. MILNE, M.S., R.D.

CONTENTS

INTRODUCTION

Have you ever walked into a drug store, pharmacy, or even a supermarket, observed the shelves and shelves of vitamin and mineral supplements, and wondered, "Who buys all of these vitamins? Are Americans *really* so undernoursihed that they need to take all these vitamin-mineral concentrates? Hmmm, I wonder if *I* should be taking something."

If these abundant displays of vitamin preparations don't convince you that you're undernourished, television advertising for such supplements may turn you into a "vitamin-pill popper." Have you ever heard, "I love my husband, and I love myself. That's why I take . . . ." Or what about, "Do you know what mineral is most important to a woman? It's iron . . . ." With so many psychological appeals being used in mass-media advertising, many Americans *must* believe they are malnourished.

What is malnutrition? Does it exist in the United States today? If so, where? What can I, as a nurse, do to help prevent or alleviate malnutrition? These questions and others will be answered in the following Activities.

PREREQUISITES FOR THIS MODULE

1. Chapters on vitamins, minerals, and deficiency diseases from one of the textbooks listed in the References for the first module. You are responsible for applying the knowledge from these chapters while completing the Activities. Be sure that you pass the Pretest and understand the rationale for the answers before preceeding to the Activities.

2. Bower, F., ed. "Nursing Assessment." *Wiley Nursing Concept Module*. New York: John Wiley & Sons, Inc., 1977. Completion of this module will help the student comprehend the scope of the Activities planned in the present module.

TERMINAL OBJECTIVES

Upon the completion of this module, the learner will be able to

1. Define *malnutrition* and *iatrogenic malnutrition.*

2. Identify deficiency symptoms for specified vitamins and minerals.

3. List the high-risk population groups for developing malnutrition.

4. List the federally funded nutrition programs designed to prevent or alleviate malnutrition.

5. Identify possible causes of iatrogenic malnutrition.

6. List the complicating physiological effects of iatrogenic malnutrition.

7. Identify the nurse's role in preventing iatrogenic malnutrition.

8. List the components of a nutritional assessment.

PRETEST

Please complete the following pretest. If you can correctly answer 80% of the questions, you may proceed to the next module, as you have demonstrated knowledge of this module. If you cannot correctly answer at least 80% of the questions, proceed to page 55.

Match the term with the correct definition.

Term	Definition
1. ___ Anorexia	a. A state of ill health, malnutrition, and wasting.
2. ___ Ascites	b. Softening of the bones, chiefly in adults
3. ___ Atrophy	c. Inflammation of the tongue
4. ___ Bitot's spots	d. Loss of appetite
5. ___ Cachetic	e. Deficiency disease related primarily to protein lack and seen in severely malnourished children
6. ___ Cheilosis	f. Abnormal drying of the skin and eyes
7. ___ Dental caries	g. Decay of the teeth
8. ___ Follicular hyperkeratosis	h. Overgrowth of the horny layer of the epidermis
9. ___ Glossitis	i. Accumulation of fluid in the abdominal cavity
10. ___ Goiter	j. Gray, shiny spots on the conjunctiva resulting from malnutrition
11. ___ Kwashiorkor	k. A deficiency disease of the skeletal system, often resulting in bone deformities
12. ___ Nyctalopia	l. Enlargement of the thyroid gland

13. ___ Osteomalacia	m.	Night-blindness; a condition in which a person cannot see well in a faint light or at night.
14. ___ Pallor	n.	Lesions of the lips and angles of the mouth
15. ___ Rickets	o.	Lack of normal tone or strength
16. ___ Xerosis	p.	Lack of color of the skin; paleness

Choose the correct answer.

17. ___ A precursor of vitamin A may be found in plants in the form of

    a) Calciferol.
    b) Carotene.
    c) Menadione.
    d) Tryptophan.

18. ___ In comparison with water-soluble vitamins, fat-soluble vitamins are

    a) More likely to be dissolved by freezing.
    b) Relatively unstable when exposed to temperatures required for microwave cooking.
    c) Less likely to be lost by ordinary cooking methods.
    d) More prone to be lost in the evaporation process.

19. ___ A vitamin that can be synthesized in the lower portion of the gastrointestinal tract by the bacterial flora is

    a) Vitamin A.
    b) Vitamin D.
    c) Vitamin E.
    d) Vitamin K.

20. ___ The vitamin that is necessary for the formation of rhodopsin, the pigment important in visual adaptation to darkness, is

a) Ascorbic acid.
b) Vitamin D.
c) Thiamin.
d) Vitamin A.

21. ___ The vitamin that has erroneously been called the "sex" vitamin in the news media is

a) Vitamin A.
b) Vitamin B_{12}.
c) Vitamin E.
d) Vitamin K.

22. ___ Hypervitaminosis is not likely to result under normal conditions but could possibly occur with

a) Ascorbic acid.
b) Vitamin D.
c) Niacin.
d) Pyridoxine.

23. ___ Rich sources of vitamin A are

a) Liver, cauliflower, and turnips.
b) Liver, tomatoes, and carrots.
c) Milk, green beans, and grits.
d) Eggs, potatoes, and salmon bones.

24. ___ A very good source of riboflavin is

a) Bananas.
b) Citrus fruits.
c) Legumes.
d) Milk.

25. ___ In the process of canning foods, which of these vitamins will be lost in the *greatest* quantities?

a) Vitamin A and vitamin C.
b) Vitamin C and thiamin.
c) Vitamin D and folic acid.
d) Vitamin K and niacin.

26. ___ The only B vitamin that is effective in curing both the symptoms of insufficient red blood cell formation and the involvement of the nervous tissue in pernicious anemia is

a) Vitamin B_6.
b) Vitamin B_{12}.
c) Riboflavin.
d) Thiamin.

27. ___ Of the following, the two vegetables that are highest in vitamin C per average serving are

a) Cabbage and potatoes.
b) Carrots and cabbage.
c) Green peas and carrots.
d) Potatoes and green peas.

28. ___ The mineral that, when present in the proportion of one part per million parts of water, has been proven effective in preventing dental decay is

a) Chlorine.
b) Fluorine.
c) Magnesium.
d) Sodium.

29. ___ Comparing the daily calcium requirement (RDA) for healthy adults, the requirement for the male is

a) Somewhat greater than for the female.
b) The same as for the female.
c) Somewhat less than for the female.
d) Substantially less than for the female.

30. ___ The daily iodine requirement is *highest* for which of these persons?

a) Infants
b) Adolescent males
c) Nonpregnant females
d) Adults 65 years of age and older

31. ___ The chief cation of intracellular fluid is

a) Calcium.
b) Magnesium.
c) Potassium.
d) Sodium.

32. ___ The mineral most often associated with edema is

a) Potassium in the extracellular fluids.
b) Sodium in the interstitial spaces.
c) Potassium in the intercellular fluids.
d) Sodium in the lymph fluids.

33. ___ Which two foods are *both* rich sources of potassium?

a) Cooked rice and fortified margarine
b) Boiled potatoes and apple juice
c) Bananas and orange juice
d) Cranberry juice and grape juice

34. ___ The relationship between vitamin D and the absorption of calcium is similar to the relationship between the intrinsic factor and the absorption of

a) Ascorbic acid.
b) Vitamin B_6.
c) Vitamin B_{12}.
d) Thiamin.

35. ___ If the diet of an infant consists mainly of milk, which of these conditions is the child likely to develop?

a) Anemia
b) Diarrhea
c) Eczema
d) Tetany

36. ___ Long-term deficiency of which of these nutrients results in goiter?

a) Iodine
b) Iron
c) Magnesium
d) Sodium

37. ___ Deficiency of ascorbic acid in the diet may produce which of these clinical symptoms?

a) Cardiac insufficiency and poor eye-hand coordination.
b) Easy bruising, poor healing of wounds, and bleeding gums
c) Incomplete digestion of carbohydrate and fat
d) Keratinization of the skin and darkening of the skin

38. ___ The vitamin whose deficiency, beriberi, produces involvement of the gastrointestinal system, the nervous system, and the cardiovascular system is

a) Niacin.
b) Pyridoxine.
c) Riboflavin.
d) Thiamin.

39. ___ Four nutrients needed for bone growth are

a) Ascorbic acid, vitamin D, fluorine, and magnesium
b) Calcium, potassium, vitamin A, and vitamin K.
c) Phosphorus, calcium, vitamin D, and magnesium
d) Thiamin, calcium, riboflavin, and iron

40. ___ Two nutrients that, in addition to iron, are especially important in promoting red blood cell formation are

a) Ascorbic acid and vitamin D.
b) Folic acid and Vitamin B_{12}.
c) Vitamin A and folic acid.
d) Vitamin A and vitamin E.

ANSWERS

1. d	3. o	5. a	7. g
2. i	4. j	6. n	8. h

9. c	17. b	25. b	33. c
10. l	18. c	26. b	34. c
11. e	19. d	27. a	35. a
12. m	20. d	28. b	36. a
13. b	21. c	29. b	37. b
14. p	22. b	30. b	38. d
15. k	23. b	31. c	39. c
16. f	24. d	32. b	40. b

ACTIVITY 1
A DEFINITION OF MALNUTRITION IN THE UNITED STATES

Among the beliefs about malnutrition that Americans have held over the past decades are the following:

1. *Malnutrition* is a *lack of* vital nutrients in the body, or an improper absorption and distribution of them, resulting in deficiency diseases, stunted growth, and/or mental retardation.

2. Malnutrition occurs only in underdeveloped or developing countries such as those of Africa, Asia, and Central America.

3. Owing to the affluence in the United States, people living in this country are immune to diseases of malnutrition.

What are the facts?

1. Today, the medical profession uses the term *malnutrition* to refer to either an overabundance or a lack of vital nutrients in the body. Therefore, the term refers to a broad spectrum of

of disease states, ranging from obesity caused by overeating to cachexia which results from cancer.

2. The Ten State Nutrition Survey and the HANES Report (refer to Module 1) revealed that every disease of malnutrition that exists in the underdeveloped countries exists also in the United States. These surveys, conducted on people living in low-income areas, found malnutrition to be most prevalent among infants, children, pregnant teenage females, and the elderly. The most common problems seen were iron-deficiency anemia, dental problems, retarded growth in children one to three years of age, vitamin A deficiency, deficiencies of vitamin B_6 (pyridoxine) and folic acid, endemic goiter, ascorbic acid (vitamin C) deficiency, vitamin D deficiency, calcium deficiency, and protein malnutrition (kwashiorkor and marasmus). When these findings were reported, numerous Senate investigations and national conferences were conducted to investigate the best means of alleviating malnutrition in the United States. As a result, new federally funded nutrition programs were started and those in existence were upgraded and expanded (see Module 1). Continued nutritional studies have proven that these programs are helping to diminish the state of malnutrition in the low-income groups.

3. The affluent middle- and upper-income classes are not without their malnourished disease states. Money does not guarantee that one eats, or knows how to eat, properly. Many of the problems in these income levels result from nutritional excesses: obesity, atherosclerosis, hypertension, cardiovascular disease--many of this country's major health diseases, as discussed in the first module. For the most part, these overnourished (not undernourished) people are the ones who purchase the vitamin-mineral supplements.

If the Dietary Goals discussed in the first module are not revised and passed by Congress, it would appear that one of the best primary prevention measures for all income levels would be to make nutrition education mandatory from kindergarten through grade 12.

Since most of the readers of this module will be involved in nursing in hospitals or long-term care facilities, the remaining activities will be devoted to iatrogenic malnutrition and nursing measures to prevent it.

PROGRESS CHECK

Answer True or False to the following questions.

1. _____ Malnutrition is defined only as a lack of vital nutrients in the body or the improper absorption and distribution of them.

2. _____ Malnutrition can occur in any income bracket.

3. _____ Malnutrition among the low-income population is most prevalent in middle-aged adults and the elderly.

4. _____ Many Americans suffer at least borderline deficiencies of iron, iodine, vitamins A and D, ascorbic acid, folic acid, and pyridoxine.

5. _____ Federally funded nutrition programs such as WIC and the Title VII Nutrition Program were started to help alleviate malnutrition in the low-income, high-risk group.

Considering the vitamin-mineral deficiencies and nutritional excess states listed in this activity, match the following nutrients with the disease states. There may be more than one answer.

	Nutrient	Disease State
6. _____	Vitamin A deficiency	a. Anemia
7. _____	Ascorbic acid deficiency	b. Atherosclerosis
8. _____	Calcium deficiency	c. Bitot's spots
9. _____	Caloric deficiency	d. Cachexia
10. _____	Caloric excess	e. Goiter
11. _____	Cholesterol excess	f. Hypertension
12. _____	Vitamin D deficiency	g. Kwashiorkor
13. _____	Folic acid deficiency	h. Marasmus
14. _____	Iodine deficiency	i. Night-blindness
15. _____	Iron deficiency	j. Obesity
16. _____	Protein deficiency	k. Osteomalacia
17. _____	Protein excess	l. Retarded growth
18. _____	Pyridoxine deficiency	m. Rickets
19. _____	Sodium excess	n. Scorbutic gums

20. What can you, as a citizen of the United States, do to help alleviate and prevent malnutrition in this country?

ANSWERS

1. False	8. k, l, m	15. a
2. True	9. d, h	16. d, g, h
3. False	10. j	17. b, f, j
4. True	11. b	18. a
5. True	12. k, m	19. f
6. c, i	13. a	
7. a, n	14. e	

20. Support legislation for federally funded nutrition programs.

    Write to your congressmen to support mandatory nutrition education in grades K through 12 and to support heading such a program with a qualified nutrition educator.

Activity 2

IATROGENIC MALNUTRITION

Iatrogenic malnutrition is defined as physician- or hospital-induced malnutrition. Recent surveys have reported that in certain hospitals from one-fourth to one-half of the medical and surgical patients who require hospitalization for two weeks or more developed protein-calorie malnutrition (PCM). Medical science is finally realizing after many years that--along with fluid and electrolyte therapy, drug therapy, blood gases, and so on--an adequate supply of protein and calories is necessary for the patient's recovery. How do hospitals induce iatrogenic malnutrition and what effect does it have on the patient?

No medical professional would purposely induce PCM, the primary form of iatrogenic malnutrition. However, the nutritional status of the patient may be endangered by not checking to see what the patient consumes from his meal trays and how well he tolerates his diet; by not weighing the patient daily; by failing to take a nutritional assessment of the patient; and by frequently withholding food pre- or post-operatively or for tests, x-rays, or drug therapy. PCM can also be the result of stress or anxiety secondary to drug or radiation therapy.

In a symposium on "Malnutrition in the Hospital," Dr. George Blackburn, one of the first physicians to investigate the causes and effects of PCM, listed the following as complicating effects of chronic malnutrition or PCM:

Progressive weakness and apathy, leading to delayed physical rehabilitation.

Depressed cell-mediated immunity, leading to increased infection, particularly gram-negative sepsis, pneumonitis, urinary tract infection, and increased wound infections impairing wound healing.

Depressed ventilatory response to hypoxia.

Increased sensitivity, and thus decreased response, to chemo- and radiotherapy.

Increased difficulty with fluid, electrolyte, and acid-base balance.

Delayed discharge and therefore more medical expenses.[1]

Let's follow a patient from the time of admission to see how PCM could develop.

G.K., a 31-year-old male, married, father of three, is a certified public accountant who opened a private practice two months ago. He was admitted to the hospital through the emergency room after an automobile accident. Because of profuse internal bleeding, G.K. had to be rushed to surgery for a total gastrectomy, and the medical history was not completed. Immediately after surgery, the patient was given two units of blood to replace that lost from the internal injury and during surgery. The postoperative orders were for 1 liter of 5% dextrose in water every 12 hours (1 L D_5W q 12 hr). The patient could receive nothing by mouth. Owing to postsurgical complications--infection at the surgical site, pneumonia, high fever, and respiratory distress--G.K.'s orders were not changed for 14 days, by which time he had developed protein-calorie malnutrition. What could have been done to prevent this?

1. A complete medical history should have been obtained from G.K.'s wife or another member of his family. Hopefully, it would have revealed that the patient had lost 15 pounds over the past two months, owing to the stress of opening up his own office. His weight on admission was 137 pounds (62.3 kilograms). He is a man of small frame, 6 feet tall, which means that he was 10% below his ideal body weight[2] and so he should be considered underweight.

2. To his underweight condition, add the stress of the accident, surgery, hospitalization, and

---

[1] "Malnutrition in the Hospital," in *Dialogues in Nutrition*, Health Learning Systems, Inc., Bloomfield, N.J., June 1977.

[2] "Desirable Weights for Men and Women," Metropolitan Life Insurance Company, 1960.

continued worrying about the new office, and we see that the body is no longer in a state of homeostasis. The endocrine system, in response to the stress, is secreting more glucagon and epinephrine and other hormones, which

a. draw on the muscle and hepatic glycogen,

b. increase catabolism of body protein and increase synthesis or urea, and

c. accelerate the breakdown of fat, resulting in ketogenesis.

The major reason for the catabolism of the body tissues at this time is the body's need for a source of glucose. Lab values expected under these conditions would be an elevation in serum glucose, urea nitrogen, and creatinine (indicating muscle breakdown); decreased serum protein and albumin; and increased ketones in the urine. The abnormal lab values should indicate to the reader that tissue catabolism is taking place and that the patient needs sufficient carbohydrate and protein to reverse this process.

3. Was the order of 1 L D_5W q 12 hr adequate, considering the metabolic processes going on with the stress of trauma and infection? G.K. was receiving only 100 g dextrose/carbohydrate or 400 Calories in the intravenous fluid. See the problem calculated below.

Problem: How many Calories was G.K. obtaining in 24 hours when the IV order was 1 L D_5W q 12 hr?

Solution: You need to know:

(1) D_5W means there are 5 g dextrose per 100 cc fluid.

(2) There are 1000 cc per liter.

(3) There are 4 Cal per gram of carbohydrate.

Let X equal carbohydrate intake per day.

$$\frac{5\text{ g}}{100\text{ cc}} = \frac{X}{2000\text{ cc (in 24 hr)}}$$

$$100\ X = 10{,}000$$

$$X = 100\text{ g carbohydrate}$$

$$\text{Cal intake in 24 hr} = (100\text{ g})\times(4\text{ Cal/g})$$

$$= 400\text{ Cal}$$

Considering his body size, stress level, and lack of physical activity, G.K. is probably expending about 2600 Calories in 24 hours, with 480 of those calories, or 120 g, being supplied by protein.[3] Probably when G.K. contracted pneumonia and spiked a high fever, the doctors were so concerned with starting antibiotic therapy that they didn't realize the importance of increasing G.K.'s nutritional intake.

Based on his caloric needs and his caloric intake, how much weight would you expect G.K. to have lost in the 14 days on IV therapy?

Problem: G.K. requires 2600 Cal/day and for 14 days has been receiving only 400 Cal/24 hr. How much weight loss could be expected in 14 days?

Solution: You need to know:

(1) There are 3500 Cal/lb of body fat.

$$\text{Cal lost each day} = 2600\text{ Cal} - 400\text{ Cal}$$

$$= 2200\text{ Cal/day}$$

---

[3]"Nutrition in Stress and Starvation," in *Dialogues in Nutrition*, Health and Learning Systems, Inc., Bloomfield, N.J., September, 1976.

$$\text{Total Cal lost} = (2200\ \text{Cal/day}) \times (14\ \text{days})$$

$$= 30{,}800\ \text{Cal}$$

$$\text{Pounds lost} = \frac{30{,}800\ \text{Cal}}{3500\ \text{Cal/lb}}$$

$$= 8.8\ \text{lb}$$

G.K. lost 8.8 lb, or 4 kg, which brought his weight down to 128.2 lb (58.3 kg). This loss of lean body weight, when his body could not afford it, was reflected at the end of the 14 days not only by an emaciated appearance, but also by low serum creatinine levels, indicating that the muscle tissue was nearly depleted. What nutritional therapy should have been suggested for G.K.? Probably 100 to 150 g glucose during the first 48 hours; thereafter, a more effective therapy to prevent tissue breakdown would have been to give amino acids along with the glucose via the peripheral vein--that is, intravenously. Some physicians are also using the intravenous fat emulsions for peripheral infusion as a means of getting in more Calories in a smaller volume. (Remember that there are only 4 Cal/g for carbohydrate and protein, but there are 9 Cal/g for fat.) G.K. should also be receiving vitamins and minerals through his IV daily, since his needs for these nutrients have also been increased with stress.

4. If bowel sounds had been heard and G.K. was not nauseated, he could have been started on oral feedings and then progressed to the postgastrectomy diets.

5. Any medications that G.K. was receiving should have been considered for possible nutrient side-effects. (Refer to March's *Handbook*, listed among the References.

6. G.K.'s weight should have been taken daily, so that if the weight loss was not immediately

apparent to anyone on the medical team, it would have been noticed in the medical record.

Many of the steps that could have been taken to prevent the PCM from developing were nursing measures. Why and how they should be taken will be covered in Activity 3.

PROGRESS CHECK

Answer True or False to the following questions.

1. _____ Iatrogenic malnutrition can be defined as hospital- or physician-induced malnutrition.

2. _____ Supplying the patient with adequate Calories and protein is not nearly as important as monitoring fluids and electrolytes, drugs, and blood gases.

3. _____ A state of malnutrition can have adverse effects on the patient's immune system, causing increased incidence of infection and prolonged hospitalization.

4. _____ Stress triggers the release of increased amounts of glucagon and epinephrine, which promote tissue synthesis.

5. _____ Laboratory indications of protein and fat tissue catabolism would be elevated serum glucose, urea nitrogen, and creatinine; decreased serum protein and albumin; and increased ketones in the urine.

6. _____ A patient receiving 1 L $D_{10}W$ q 8 hr would be receiving 1200 Calories in 24 hours.

7. _____ If intravenous triglycerides were used to supply the number of Calories administered in question 6, one would have to administer only 1.5 liters in 24 hours.

8. _____ There are no known interactions between medications and nutrients.

9. _____ Nutritional assessment is a one-time process to be conducted only at the time of admission.

10. _____ Nutritional assessment should include physical examination, laboratory values, drugs, and a verbal dietary history.

ANSWERS

1. True
2. False
3. True
4. False
5. True
6. True
7. True
8. False
9. False
10. True

ACTIVITY 3

THE NURSE AS A MEMBER OF THE NUTRITION SUPPORT TEAM

"Why the nurse?" you say to yourself. "Why should I have to be bothered with the patient's nutritional status? I'm already overburdened. I thought dietitians were responsible for seeing to the nutritional well-being of the patients. And what about the physician?"

Time studies have shown that the floor nurse has more contact hours with her assigned patients than does the dietitian or physician. This is not to absolve either of those parties from his or her responsibilities in maintaining the nutritional status of the patient. But the nurse, as part of her ordinary routine, can do a nutritional assessment while she is completing the standard admitting nursing notes. Including the following points in the admitting notes or nursing history should help the nurse and other members of the health-care team determine the patient's nutritional status and alert them to any possible problems.

1. Height.

2. Present weight. (Actually weigh the patient; do not record what the patient "says" he weighs unless obtaining a weight is impossible. In that case, be certain to record that it is a "stated" and not an actual weight.)

3. Any recent weight gains or losses.

4. Presence of dentures, oral appliances. How do they fit?

5. Food likes? Dislikes? Allergies?

6. Eating patterns--times, places, amount in a typical day (including liquids).

7. Alcohol use? How much? Tobacco use? How much?

8. Any problems with chewing? Swallowing? Heartburn? Belching? Nausea?

9. Physical appearance (for example, obese, skinny, teeth discolored, pallor).

10. Use of therapeutic diets (such as sodium-controlled, diabetic).

11. Elimination patterns--frequency, consistency, color, odor, gas, pain, constipation, diarrhea.

12. Activity level at home (such as bed rest versus working and active.

13. Home situation--cooking facilities, socioeconomic factors, family, religion, ethnic group.

14. Past operations? Past hospitalizations?

15. Any medications? (Include vitamins, antacids, aspirin, and the like.)

The following is an example of the findings from a nutritional history[4] and how the nurse can make a nutritional assessment from it.

SAMPLE NUTRITIONAL HISTORY
Taken from Hospital Admitting Notes

Name: Mr. P.M. Age: 74 years Sex: Male

1. Height: 5'11" (177 cm)
2. Present Weight: 132 lb (60 kg)

   Normal Weight: 154 lb (70 kg) Stated by patient.
3. Lost 22 lb (10 kg) in the past two months, patient statement.
4. Upper and lower dentures that fit loosely as a result of weight loss.
5. Likes all foods. "It's been hard to eat with my dentures slipping. I must eat softer foods now with my dentures and diarrhea." Allergic to nuts, shellfish, coconut, chocolate.
6. Breakfast--0600
   - 1 c oatmeal with 1 tsp sugar, ¼ c whole milk
   - 2 slices white toast with 1 tsp margarine on each
   - 2 c black coffee

   Lunch--1200
   - ½ c cottage cheese
   - 2 canned peach halves
   - 1 glass water

   Dinner--1700
   - 1 c macaroni and cheese (frozen, heated up)
   - ½ c applesauce
   - 2 c tea with 1 tsp sugar in each

[4]For background on taking a nursing history, refer to Bower's "Nursing Assessment," listed in the Prerequisites for this module.

"I know I should be eating better, but I don't have much energy to fix much food. Nothing tastes very good right now when I know I'll be losing it in a few hours."

7. Does not use alcohol or tobacco..

8. Problems with chewing and keeping dentures in place.

9. Thin; bones are prominent with some decubiti forming on the pressure points; pale; lethargic; dry skin and hair; numerous bruses.

10. No history of therapeutic diet.

11. Stools--"4 to 5 per day for the past two months, very loose, black, foul odor"; no pain on elimination.

12. Inactive, stays in room; very weak; afraid to go beyond living quarters with diarrhea.

13. Lives in an efficiency retirement apartment partially federally funded; a widower; no children; stove/oven, sink with running water, refrigerator; the apartment provides a housekeeper to come in once a week to clean; receiving pension and social security.

14. No previous operations or hospitalization.

15. No medications, vitamins, antacids, aspirin.

The nurse, besides completing the nutritional history form, can summarize her findings in a couple of paragraphs in the nursing notes, or she can SOAP chart the information if the problem-oriented medical record (POMR) is used in her facility. Let's see how the above information can be summarized in SOAP charting form.

SOAP Chart

Subjective:

Patient states he has lost 10 kg in the past two months because of severe diarrhea and no appetite. "Nothing tastes very good right now when I know I'll be losing it in a few hours." He states the stools are loose, black, and have a foul odor. "It's been hard to eat with my dentures slipping. I know I should be eating better, but I don't have much energy to fix much food."

Objective:

Very thin--5'11", 132 lb, therefore 26 lb (16%) below ideal body weight.[5]

Decubiti forming on pressure points, numerous bruises.

Poorly fitting dentures.

Stool specimen is dark, tarry.

Assessment:

Cachetic, possible Protein-Calorie Malnutrition.

From stated dietary recall, the patient's diet is deficient in all the Basic Four Food Groups except the bread and cereal group.

Plans:

Order a dietary consult to do a more thorough nutritional assessment, including anthropometric measurements.[6]

Suggest a high-Calorie, high-protein, mechanical soft diet with 6-7 small feedings a day after diarrhea is under control. Until the diarrhea stops, suggest 7 cans of Sustacal q 24 hr, alternating flavors to meet patient's likes.

[5]"Desirable Weights for Men and Women," Metropolitan Life Insurance Company, 1960.

[6]A good source of information about anthropometric measurements is Howard and Herbold's *Nutrition in Clinical Care*, listed in the References.

Plans: (continued)

Multivitamin supplement.

Ascorbic acid.

Hold iron medication until the etiology of the dark, tarry stools has been determined.

The nutritional assessment, completed and charted by the nurse, is her form of communication with the other members of the medical team. Unless she is a nurse clinician with authority to write orders, it is now up to the physician to write the orders, arrange for a diet consult and tests, and so on.

It would be ideal if every patient in the hospital could be nutritionally assessed by a dietitian. Unfortunately, very few hospitals have budgets large enough to hire the number of dietitians that this would require. For this reason, and because doctors are graduating from medical school with very little knowledge about nutrition, the nurse's role in assessing the nutritional status of the patient is all the more important.

The nutritional assessment does not end with the admitting notes. It is an ongoing process to include laboratory and other test findings; assessment of physical, mental, and emotional status; and medications and other treatments. For example, P.M.'s laboratory analyses came back, and all of the following serum constituents were well below normal: albumin, hemoglobin, hematocrit, calcium, magnesium, potassium, and sodium. Because the attending physician had made rounds previously, he wanted the nurse to call him to report any abnormal lab values so that he could write the appropriate orders. In this case, the physician wrote an order for 1 unit of packed red blood cells, 1 liter Ringers Lactate q 12 hr, and a mineral supplement. When the nurse started the blood and the IV, she noticed that there was prolonged bleeding at both sites where the needles were injected. She charted this so that the doctor could order a prothrombin time to be run or order a vitamin K supplement if need be. P.M. was also scheduled for a lower GI x-ray, which meant that he had to go without oral nutritional support overnight. Therefore, the nurse made certain that he received a tray of allowed nourishing liquids after he had rested a while following the x-ray.

As another part of the nutrition assessment, the nurse checks the patient's meal trays, charting how well he has eaten. She also checks his emotional attitude about the food and whether his elimination habits and physical appearance have improved over what was stated in the admitting notes. All of these factors are important in the ongoing nutritional assessment. Sometimes we get so overburdened with our tasks of the moment, such as starting an IV or emptying a bedpan, that we forget to take note of all the physical cues (bleeding at the injection site, consistency of stool, appearance of the skin, and so on) that could give insight to the patient's nutritional status. Those cues *must* be observed and recorded by the nurse to help prevent iatrogenic malnutrition from occurring in her patients.

Without the nurse's observations and assessments, the physician and dietitian have little information with which to work. The nurse is definitely a vital member of the nutrition support team.

PROGRESS CHECK

1. Relate Mr. M.'s elimination problems to his laboratory analyses.

2. Relate Mr. M.'s living conditions to his eating habits.

3. Briefly summarize what should be included in a nutritional assessment.

ANSWERS

1. Decreased hemoglobin and hematocrit could be the result of internal bleeding, showing up in the black stools. The loss of electrolytes, Ca, and Mg is due to the diarrhea and fluid loss.

2. P.M. may not eat well because he eats alone. Investigate the possibility of a Title VII Program in P.M.'s living vicinity to increase socialization during at least one meal a day. Also investigate the possibility of his receiving Meals-On-Wheels when he goes home until he is stronger.

3. a. Past and present food intake, habits, likes, dislikes, allergies.

   b. Lifestyle--socioeconomic status, environment.

   c. Any handicapping conditions, physical or mechanical.

   d. Weight history.

e. Physical assessment, including emotional assessment.

f. Laboratory and other test results.

g. Medications and treatments.

SUMMARY

Malnutrition is a worldwide health problem. It escapes no country or income group. Though you may see isolated cases of vitamin deficiency diseases in your nursing practice, protein-calorie malnutrition is what you will most frequently be dealing with in hospital and long-term care facilities. In order to learn to take a good nutritional history on a patient as a part of the nursing history, you will need to practice. Practice on friends and relatives. And as you are walking down the street, waiting for a bus, or sitting in a restaurant, practice doing observational nutritional assessments on people so that the "cues" you need to be aware of become inherent in your thought process.

POSTTEST

1. ___ Deficiency of ascorbic acid in the diet may produce these clinical symptoms:

   a) Cardiac insufficiency and poor eye-hand coordination.
   b) Easy bruising, poor healing of wounds, and bleeding gums.
   c) Incomplete digestion of carbohydrate and fats.
   d) Keratinization of the skin and darkening of the skin.

2. ___ Two nutrients besides iron that are especially important in promoting red blood cell formation are

a) Ascorbic acid and vitamin D.
b) Folic acid and vitamin B_{12}.
c) Vitamin A and folic acid.
d) Vitamin A and vitamin E.

3. ___ Deficiency of vitamin K, either in the diet or induced by severe diarrhea, may produce these clinical symptoms:

a) Abnormal drying of the skin and hair.
b) Easy bruising and prolonged blood clotting time.
c) Night-blindness.
d) Weakness and pallor.

4. ___ Which of the following statements pertaining to malnutrition are *TRUE*?

1) Malnutrition is defined as an overabundance or lack of vital nutrients in the body.
2) Malnutrition can occur in any income bracket.
3) Malnutrition among the low-income population is most prevalent in middle-aged adults and the elderly.
4) Many Americans suffer at least borderline deficiencies of iodine; calcium; iron; vitamins A, C, D, folic acid, and B_6 (pyridoxine).

Choose the correct answer from among the following:

a) 1, 2, and 3
b) 1, 2, and 4
c) 1, 3, and 4
d) 2, 3, and 4

5. ___ Iatrogenic malnutrition can have which of the following adverse effects?

1) Progressive weakness and apathy.
2) Increased infection.

3) Decreased difficulty with fluid, electrolyte, and acid-base balance.
4) Delayed physical rehabilitation and discharge.

Choose the correct answer from among the following:

a) 1, 2, and 3
b) 1, 2, and 4
c) 1, 3, and 4
d) 2, 3, and 4

6. ___ Laboratory indications of tissue catabolism would include

1) Decreased serum glucose.
2) Increased serum urea nitrogen and creatinine.
3) Decreased serum protein and albumin.
4) Decreased ketones in the urine.

Choose the correct answer from among the following:

a) 1 and 2
b) 1 and 4
c) 2 and 3
d) 3 and 4

7. ___ A patient receiving 1 L D_5W q 8 hr would be receiving how many Calories in 24 hours?

a) 200
b) 400
c) 600
d) 800

8. ___ The patient in question 7 is under the stress of having had surgery and requires 2400 Calories per day. If he receives IV therapy as the sole source of Calories for one week, approximately how much weight would you expect him to lose in that week?

a) 3.0 lb
b) 3.5 lb
c) 4.0 lb
d) 4.5 lb

9. ___ A nutritional assessment should include which of the following?

1) Dietary history
2) Physical assessment
3) Laboratory and test results
4) Medications and other therapy

Choose the correct answer from among the following:

a) 1 only
b) 1 and 2
c) 1, 2, and 3
d) 1, 2, 3, and 4

ANSWERS

1. b
2. b
3. b
4. b
5. b
6. c
7. c
8. b
9. d

REFERENCES

Butterworth, C.E. and G.L. Blackburn. "Hospital Nutrition." *Nutrition Today*, 10: 2 (March/April 1975).

Howard, R. and N. Herbold. *Nutrition in Clinical Care*. New York: McGraw-Hill, 1978.

"Malnutrition in the Hospital." *Dialogues in Nutrition*. Bloomfield, N.J.: Health Learning Systems, Inc., June 1977.

March, D.C. *Handbook: Interactions of Selected Drugs with Nutritional Status in Man.* Chicago: The American Dietetic Association, 1976.

"Nutrition in Stress and Starvation." *Dialogues in Nutrition.* Bloomfield, N.J.: Health Learning Systems, Inc., September 1976.

Internal and External Factors Affecting Food Consumption

PEGGY STANFIELD, M.S., R.D.

CONTENTS

INTRODUCTION

Feelings, attitudes, conditioning, and economics continually affect one's food consumption throughout life. Except for health professionals, who are well aware of the vital role nutrition plays in the maintenance of health and the recovery from illness, most people give these aspects of food priority over its importance for health.

Culture is a way of life. It is useful in adapting a person to his environment. Beginning with his very earliest experiences, the child acquires customs and attitudes which he begins to internalize. Along with his food, he receives information that affects his feelings and values; these remain on a subconscious level and are therefore very difficult to change. Eating habits, then, develop as a complex pattern of feelings, values, attitudes, and customary behavior.

Economics is a very strong factor in the determination of food consumption. The costs of producing, transporting, and distributing food determine how much and what types of food are available. Lack of money affects not only the prices that people can pay for food, but also the kinds of storage facilities they can afford to have within the household. People in poverty must buy cheaper foods in smaller quantities and must limit purchases to items that do not require special storage facilities such as freezers or refrigerators. The cost of transportation may make traveling to a larger market, where volume buying enables the merchant to sell more cheaply, economically unrealistic for some impoverished consumers. Poverty is sometimes classified as a subculture in our society, and from it emerge different attitudes and adaptations about foods than are found in the middle or upper classes. Nurses need extensive knowledge of these differences.

Eating is generally engaged in because of hunger or appetite. Hunger is a physiological mechanism controlled by the central nervous system. It is an unpleasant sensation. Appetite is a desire for food related to past experiences in response to stimuli such as smell, taste, and appearance. Appetite is not necessarily related to biological needs. People who are really hungry will eat many things not within their cultural frame of reference. They adapt physiologically and psychologically in order to prolong survival. Appetite, on the other hand, can become uncontrolled behavior and result in obesity, which is also a form of malnutrition since there is usually a deficiency of some essential nutrients.

The biological food needs of a person throughout the life cycle are only that his food provide him with essential chemical substances--nutrients--which he can digest, absorb, and metabolize. In order to maintain life and health, the nutrients must reach the cells. Adequate nutrient intake depends on many factors, including age, sex, activity, size, and individual variations. The amounts of nutrients required may vary, but the types and kinds of nutrients established as being essential to life and health will remain the same throughout life. Research may add other, heretofore unrecognized, essentials as scientific investigation progresses.

Planned change is a deliberate intervention to bring about improvement. Some of the factors to be considered in planning changes in food habits are personal and societal values, environment, biological need, the teacher's expectations and acculturation, and decisions made by influential government agencies and industry. The planner must also take into account that change is slow; the learner will absorb only what he feels is relevant and useful to him at a given time.

Abstract knowledge is rarely sufficient in itself to motivate someone to make a change. All the scientific knowledge and reasoning that you can bring to the client's attention will have little effect unless you can relate these facts intimately to his culture and eating habits. The client will respond more favorably if you work with him in the framework of his culture, his social and psychological conditioning, and his situational dimensions. It is essential to encourage whatever good elements are found in the client's present eating pattern and to motivate him to change those elements that require change.

This module is designed to help the reader determine some of the internal and external factors factors affecting food consumption. It also offers some experience in planning therapeutic interventions when food behaviors must be changed in order to maintain or restore health.

PREREQUISITES FOR THIS MODULE

It is not necessary to have completed a course in nutrition, although a basic knowledge of normal nutrition may increase the student's understanding of the module. An approved textbook on human nutrition will aid the student in determining specific nutritional requirements at various stages of the life cycle.

TERMINAL OBJECTIVES

Upon the completion of this module, the learner will be able to:

1. Describe the cultural, social, and psychological factors that influence nutritional behavior.

    a. Distinguish between biologic necessity and cultural patterning.

    b. Identify the use of food in a culture.

    c. Explain the symbolism of food in a culture.

    d. Identify the social influences of food in a culture.

    e. Describe the psychological influence of food.

2. Determine the economic considerations that affect food intake.

3. Identify the nutritional requirements of humans at various stages of the life cycle.

4. Explain the factors that affect the potential for behavior changes in an individual's eating patterns.

5. Given data, demonstrate an ability to plan effective nutrition teaching.

PRETEST

Before beginning this module, take the following pretest. If you are able to answer 80% of the questions correctly, you need not complete this module. You may proceed to another module. The correct answers are given at the end of the test.

1. Distinguish between biologic necessity and cultural patterning.

2. Explain the following:

   a) The use of food in a culture

   b) The use of food symbolism

c) The social influences of food

3. What economic considerations affect food intake?

4. List five factors that affect the potential for behavior changes in eating patterns.

5. List six factors that should be assessed when planning health teaching.

6. Identify the information to be obtained from a diet history.

7. Explain the factor most influential in determining whether learning has occurred.

ANSWERS

1. Biologic necessity refers to the nutrient balance that the body requires in order to maintain life and health. Cultural patterning, on the other hand, establishes values, feelings, attitudes, and beliefs regarding food consumption. The required nutrient levels may or may not be met.

2. a) Food is used in a culture to adapt a person to his environment. It reflects the social organization of a people, including their religion, economy, and psychological attitudes.

   b) Food symbolism is related to security. This security can be emotional, biological, or sociological.

c) Social influences of foods denote status, acceptance, roles in life, and class structure.

3. The cost of food production, transportation, and distribution determines how much and what types of food are available. Economics also affects food purchase, storage, and preparation. Poverty gives people different attitudes and adaptations toward food than people at other economic levels have.

4. (1) Awareness of personal and societal values.

   (2) Environment.

   (3) Biological need.

   (4) Cultural patterning, biases, and attitudes.

   (5) Legislation enacted regarding food products, such as manufacturing and labeling requirements and quality standards.

5. (1) What does the person want to learn, if anything?

   (2) Is he or is he not in crisis?

   (3) What is his definition of health and illness?

   (4) What kind of communication does he respond to? (Education level, age, language, and so on.)

   (5) What is his developmental stage?

   (6) What gives meaning to his life? (His culture, social class, religion, environment, and the like.)

6. Kinds of food that are culturally acceptable.

   Any religious restrictions.

Meals--where eaten, when, with whom?

Food preparation--by whom, facilities for storage, methods, safety.

Amount of money spent for food, kinds of food purchased.

Typical intake--a 24-hour recall, including snacks.

Food allergies, dislikes, intolerances.

Handicaps that may interfere with eating (such as lack of teeth; paralysis of arm, hand, throat, and so on).

7. If the individual adopts the proposed change and incorporates it into his daily living pattern, then it can be assumed that learning has occurred.

ACTIVITY 1

THE DEVELOPMENT OF EATING BEHAVIOR

Eating behaviors develop from cultural, societal, and psychological patterns. These patterns, reflecting food habits that have been transmitted from preceding generations, are the heritage of any given ethnic group. They may be influenced by interactions with other groups, so that some intermingling of patterns is inevitable, but modifications are worked into the total structure over long periods of time and are acceptable only if they fit the existing customs.

According to Robinson, food patterns reflect a people's social organization, including their economy, religion, beliefs about the health properties of foods, and attitudes about family. Great emotional significance is attached to the consumption of certain foods.[1]

---

[1]Robinson, C., *Normal and Therapeutic Nutrition*, (New York: Mcmillan, 1977).

Eating behaviors are derived from many sources. To become part of the eating pattern, a food must be available and acceptable within the cultural context. The ways in which a food is determined to be acceptable vary greatly among societies and among individuals, and both conscious and unconscious criteria are applied. One such criterion is food symbolism, which is the meaning attached to food. Those foods symbolically designated positive are acceptable, whereas negative evaluation causes rejection.

Most food symbolism is related to security. This security can be emotional, biological, or sociological, or any combination of the three. For instance, foods believed to have safety and health benefits offer biological security. An example is food faddism--the belief that eating certain foods will bring special health benefits.

Great numbers of food taboos and superstitions are associated with biological symbolism. Food taboos are based on beliefs that certain foods or food combinations are bad or unsafe. Superstitions arise from beliefs about magical powers of foods. For example, certain herbs are believed to ward off old age. It does not matter that there may be little or no scientific basis for these beliefs. It is what the individual thinks that influences his choice.

Nowhere is food symbolism more pronounced than in the context of emotional security. A deep emotional attachment to food begins from the moment an individual receives his first food from a significant other. Eating is associated with love, caring, attention, and satisfaction. One of the causes of obesity may be a response to this emotional association. Food may also be used for discipline, punishment, reward for moral virtue, and bribery; hence, the response elicited by such uses of certain foods may be frustration, anger, and rejection. Food is often used as a weapon or a crutch. A child learns the hidden meanings of food very quickly and will use this tool for power and manipulation--for example, refusing to eat, throwing a tantrum, or developing sudden whims. For the teenager, strenuous dieting, refusal to eat foods that are good for him, or voracious overeating are weapons that usually gain him what he wants. Used as a crutch, food becomes an emotional outlet for boredom, frustration, anxiety, and other stresses. Using food as a crutch is also a contributing factor in obesity.

Food and religion are linked symbolically with emotional security. In all religions, certain foods are used in ceremonial rites as a means of demonstrating faith and for commemorating events. Prohibition of certain foods is also common practice. Examples of religious food symbolism include Holy Communion in Christian churches, the Jewish dietary laws, and the prohibiting of the use of animal flesh by Hindus and Buddhists. Fasting is common to most religions. Often the reasons for food prohibitions are obscure.

Sociological symbolism can include the use of food as a status symbols--that is, certain foods are considered desirable because of high cost, difficulty in obtaining or preparing them, and/or superior quality. Examples include prime rib, imported wines, truffles, caviar, fancy and complicated desserts, and other such food choices. Also of sociological significance is the use of foods as a means of communication. Eating together denotes acceptance. Practically all social occasions involve food or drink. Examples include refreshments at meetings, weddings, and feasts. Dinner parties and dinner dates are socially significant. Foods communicate roles in life as loudly as do actions.

Of the various kinds of security-related food symbolism, sociological symbolism is the one most likely to change. Social meanings attached to food are not as deeply imbedded in the psyche as are emotional and biological meanings. Social symbols change as situations and experiences change.

Illness modifies food acceptance. Anxiety, loneliness, unfamiliar foods, lack of activity, and the disease process all contribute to an alteration of usual eating patterns. Appetite may diminish, and hostility or apathy about food may occur. Children may regress to an earlier developmental stage, and adults may regress to less mature states.

Some examples should help the student to understand the forces at work in the development of eating behaviors.

EXAMPLE 1

Mary W., age 65, states that she takes 2 tablespoons of lethicin, 1200 mg of organic vitamin E, plus a cup of rose hip tea each day to "keep her arteries cleared out" and "prevent arthritis."

1. What eating behavior is being manifested by Mary?

2. Is this a superstition or a taboo?

EXAMPLE 2

Jane is your roommate. The night before the final exam in anatomy and physiology, the two of you go to the store and purchase six donuts, four candy bars, a bag of popcorn, a pound of peanuts, and a carton of cola beverage because you don't plan to take time out for dinner.

3. What eating behavior are you manifesting?

4. Was the choice of foods based on scientific evidence of the need for extra energy while studying strenuously?

EXAMPLE 3

Jesus Martinez, age 35, is admitted to your floor in the hospital for lab tests tomorrow. His lunch tray contains broiled fish, asparagus, baked potato, jello, and milk. It is an attractive tray. He does not touch the food. As he speaks no English and you no Spanish, you are unable to ask about it.

5. What may you assume is the cause of this rejection?

EXAMPLE 4

Ellen confides to you that her mother once made her sit at the breakfast table for three hours until she ate her bowl of oatmeal and that she will never touch another bite of oatmeal as long as she lives. "The thought of cold, sticky, nasty oatmeal makes me want to throw up."

6. What factors are involved in Ellen's feelings about the oatmeal?

EXAMPLE 5

Mrs. Theo F. Jones III, wife of a prominent government official, is the guest of honor at a luncheon where hamburger casserole is the main entree. She barely touches any of the food and leaves immediately afterward, even though she had planned to speak on a pet project.

7. Was Mrs. Jones ill, allergic to hamburger, or angry?

8. What type of food symbolism is manifested here?

ANSWERS FOR EXAMPLES

1. Biological food symbolism. Food faddism--the belief that certain foods bring special health benefits--is very prevalent.

2. Superstition--a set of beliefs about the magical powers of food. There does not have to be a scientific basis for such beliefs.

3. Emotional food symbolism. Students' eating patterns change during exam time. They usually eat more, and the choices are usually high-Calorie items. Such eating seems to help relieve strain.

4. There is no scientific evidence of need for extra Calories while studying. One peanut would probably furnish enough energy for the entire study period.

5. There could be several causes, including anxiety, fear, unfamiliar surroundings, and strange people presenting the food, but the major cause is probably that these foods are not culturally acceptable.

6. Ellen is projecting an unpleasant memory associated with oatmeal. This frequently causes a

a food once eaten to become unacceptable. Psychotic patients often show great agitation by spitting on a food or dashing the tray to the floor when it brings back unpleasant memories. This is another example of emotional food symbolism.

7. Angry. Food is used as a status symbol, and hamburger definitely is not included among status foods. She felt rejected and humiliated by this menu. She felt it did not reflect her social standing.

8. Sociological food symbolism.

PROGRESS CHECK

Analyze *your* eating patterns. Be as objective as possible. Answer the following questions about your behaviors.

1. What are the determining factors in the way you eat?

2. What are the determining factors in the amount you eat?

3. What determines your likes and dislikes?

4. What causes a new food to be acceptable or unacceptable to you?

5. What is your favorite food? Why?

6. What are the strengths and weaknesses of your diet?

7. List the factors that determine what foods are available to you.

ACTIVITY 2

FOOD CONSUMPTION AND BIOLOGICAL WELL-BEING

A reciprocal relationship exists between food consumption and physical health. Four basic, simple nutrition concepts that the nurse can use to assess biological well-being will be briefly explored in this activity. Biological well-being may be considered a satisfactory state of physical health.

1. *The Concept of Nutrition*

   Nutrition is the food you eat and how the body uses it. Implied in this definition are many complex processes, including cultural, social, economic, religious, and individual factors that determine what is acceptable as food. How the body uses food refers to the whole metabolic process and all the factors that affect it, including biological individuality, the interrelationship among the nutrients, and heredity.

2. *The Concept of Nutrients*

   Food is made up of different nutrients. Nutrients are chemical substances. In order for the body to survive, the nutrients must be available at the cellular level. All nutrients needed by the body are available through food. Many kinds and combinations of food will provide a balanced diet. Each nutrient has specific uses in the body. No food, by itself, has all the nutrients the body needs for growth and health. The nutrients are interrelated. They are most effective when ingested together.

3. *The Concept of Enough Food*

   All persons throughout life have need for the same nutrients, but in varying amounts. The amounts vary with age, sex, size, activity, and state of health. The nutrients determined to be essential to life and health are oxygen, water, carbohydrates, proteins, fats, vitamins, and minerals. While energy is not a nutrient, but rather is the fuel source of the body contained in nutrients, it must be considered in the concept of enough food. It is measured in Calories or Joules. If a person lacks sufficient Calories, he is hungry. If he lacks one or more essential nutrients, he is malnourished. Nutrient imbalance and overnutrition are also considered forms of malnutrition.

Recommendations for the kinds and amounts of nutrients required are made by trained scientists and interpreted in terms of specific foods by nutritionists, nurses, and other health professionals. The National Academy of Science provides the Recommended Dietary Allowances, and the Basic Four Food Groups cover a range of foods that will meet these allowances.

4. *The Concept of Safe Food*

The way food is handled influences its safety, appearance, taste, and the amount of nutrients it contains. Handling includes everything that happens to food while it is being grown, processed, transported, stored, and prepared for eating. In America, stringent regulations, enforced by federal agencies, safeguard food supplies through the first four steps and also provide for inspection of public eating places for cleanliness and sanitation. In private homes, however, food safety and preparation practices are an individual matter.

PROGRESS CHECK

1. List and describe the four basic nutrition concepts.

2. Define *biological well-being*.

3. The following statement is true: "Ethnic groups with varied lifestyles and divergent eating patterns may all be able to eat a balanced diet." Briefly explain why the statement is true.

4. From what source do the recommendations for North America's essential nutrients come?

5. Which of the nutrients will furnish energy for the body?

ANSWERS

1. See the four concepts of nutrition discussed in Activity 2.
2. A satisfactory state of physical health.
3. From the concept of nutrients: All nutrients are available through food. Many kinds and combinations of food will provide a balanced diet.
4. The National Academy of Science.
5. Carbohydrates, protein, and fats. Oxygen, water, vitamins, and minerals, while essential for life and health, do not furnish energy. They are, however, directly involved in the metabolism of energy-providing nutrients.

Activity 3

FACTORS AFFECTING BEHAVIORAL CHANGES IN FOOD CONSUMPTION

The student may wonder why changes in food consumption patterns are needed, particularly in the United States. In recent years, because of better research and better interpretation of data regarding the nutritional status of individuals, it has become increasingly clear that primary malnutrition exists in the United States. It is now recognized that overnutrition, misinformation, ignorance, poor economic status, and poor eating habits are prevalent in this country. Malnutrition is very difficult to deal with in the United States because of the diverse population with its many cultures, subcultures, values, and experiences. Among the common nutritional problems are obesity, iron-deficiency anemia (especially among low-income women of childbearing age and among infants), and suboptimal intakes of calcium, ascorbic acid, and vitamin A. Special nutritional problems affect the poor, the elderly, and the adolescent. The need for change is clear.

The stages of change begin with an awareness that there is a problem. Identifying the problem and offering alternatives to the present behavior is the teaching stage. This is not a simple task. Important factors that influence behavior changes are the values, attitudes, beliefs, motivation, and knowledge level of the learner. These same factors apply to the teacher and can create barriers to successful communication unless a common frame of reference is developed. The final stage of change is preceded by a trial period with reinforcement. The expected outcome is adoption of the change.

Learning is very personal and is measured in terms of changed behavior. The basic principles of learning, focused upon the learner, are individuality, contact, listening, participation, need fulfillment, and appraisal.[2] In order to incorporate

---

[2]Williams, S.R., *Nutrition and Diet Therapy*, (St. Louis: C.V. Mosby Co., 1977).

these principles successfully, the teacher needs a broad knowledge of the habits, customs, behavior, and beliefs of the individual with whom the interaction is to occur. This knowledge will expedite understanding of the reasons for that person's food-consumption patterns. These patterns serve a useful function for the person and cannot be abruptly dismissed if communication is to continue.

Participation by the client can occur only if he is actively engaged in his own learning process. The client needs to feel free to express his concerns, to explore his feelings, to state his problems, and to help plan his care. A successful teacher is able to elicit these responses.

In order to facilitate the learning process, the teacher should become an active listener. The interview is more effective when it is of a nondirective nature. Reflection, exploratory responses (such as "go on"), restatement, and clarification all provide a supportive atmosphere, are useful tools for information gathering, and help engage the client in participation in his own learning. Offering alternatives, a more direct approach, can be used in later contacts after mutual trust is established. Appraisal of the learning that is taking place should be done by both the teacher and the learner.

PROGRESS CHECK

1. Briefly explain why there is a need to change food-consumption patterns in the United States.

2. What are the most common nutritional problems in the United States today?

3. Name one factor that starts the process of change.

4. What factors influence behavior changes?

5. What is the role of the teacher in the teaching-learning process?

6. List the basic principles of learning as focused upon the learner.

7. What technique is being used when reflection, clarification, and restatement are employed in an interview?

8. How is learning evaluated?

ANSWERS

1. There is statistical evidence of primary malnutrition in the United States.

2. Obesity, iron-deficiency anemia, suboptimal intakes of calcium and vitamins A and C. Other special problems affect the poor, the elderly, and the adolescent.

3. Awareness that there is a problem.

4. Values, attitudes, beliefs, motivation, and knowledge level.

5. The teacher is the facilitator of change. She identifies the problem and offers alternatives.

6. Individuality, contact, listening, participation, need fulfillment, and appraisal.

7. These are part of the nondirective technique of counseling. This approach involves the teacher in active listening. It proves most useful in early interviews by engaging the client in participation in his own learning.

8. Learning is measured in terms of changed behavior. Evaluation is made to determine whether the proposed changes are adapted into the client's lifestyle.

ACTIVITY 4
THE NURSE'S RESPONSIBILITY FOR HEALTH EDUCATION

Health education implies that the client will participate in his own care. In order to do this, the client must have someone teach him how. Such teaching--whether the client needs to know how to give himself and injection or how to improve his nutrition--cannot be separated from total care.

The nurse thus shares the responsibility for health education with the other members of the team responsible for the client's well-being.

Valid health education is based on the accurate statement of related facts that have been demonstrated scientifically.[3] The nurse, as part of the health team, is responsible for having a sound background knowledge of nutrition and the role it plays in bringing about other improvements in health. She must share the responsibility for nutrition education with her teammates. If she is not the primary teacher, she will support and encourage the client to follow the instructions given by another professional and will provide relevant feedback for evaluation purposes. Often she will assume the primary role because of her proximity to the client or because it is an integral part of the comprehensive health care given the client.

Whatever the area--at bedside, during a treatment, or in the community--the nurse has the opportunity to teach. The nurse should teach health promotion by example: personal hygiene, health precautions, and a positive attitude. She must consider the total person. The total person has been the thrust of this module.

A review of the factors involved in assessing the total person will facilitate the setting up of effective teaching plans:

1. What does the person want to learn, if anything?

2. Is he or is he not in crisis?

3. What is his definition of health and illness?

4. What kind of communication does he respond to? (Education level, age, language, and so on.)

5. What is his developmental stage?

6. What gives meaning to his life? (His culture, social class, religion, environment, and the like.)

---

[3]Williams, *Nutrition and Diet Therapy*, p. 297.

Since nursing students are familiar with the problem-solving process, this is the tool we will use to illustrate nutritional counseling.

Step 1: Assessment

Data gathered for assessment should include the internal and external factors that affect the client's food consumption. The questions about the six factors involved in the assessment of the total person should be answered. Any pertinent medical history should be noted. A diet history furnishes important assessment data. Not every item will be required for every client, nor will direct questioning be required for every client, but there should be enough data for a significant assessment to be made. The interview is an integral part of assessment.

Step 2: Planning

Planning can proceed from the assessment of the initial data and the identified needs. After the needs are identified, it may be necessary to research the literature in order to form an appropriate counseling plan. The nurse cannot be expected to keep a large fund of current information from all the sciences in her memory, but she should know about sources--where to locate pertinent information for a particular case and how to interpret and apply this information to the identified needs of her client. Referral agencies should be noted if needed. The counseling plan should state, in writing, clearly defined learner objectives. These objectives should be agreed upon by both the teacher and the learner. They must be realistic and specific. They must be stated in measurable terms--that is, they should be behavioral objectives. They should be related to the assessed needs of the client and relevant to the world in which he functions. They should encompass eventual client independence.

Step 3: Implementation

If the client has helped to choose the objectives in the planning stage, the implementation should proceed more smoothly. Implementation includes the presentation of the knowledge the learner needs in order to proceed with his learning and practice through the provision of learning experiences. The nursing student is well aware of the value of visual aids, demonstrations, role playing, and other such techniques which enhance learning. These and other learning strategies are useful in implementation.

Step 4: Evaluation

Evaluation measures the success of the counseling. It serves a dual purpose by indicating the success or failure of both the client's learning and the teacher's efficiency. Evaluation may include both competence and motivation. It may include recall, return demonstrations, and other techniques that show whether the client has met the objectives. If the objectives are not met, the teacher must revise her counseling plan and reapproach the client. If the client can meet the objectives, there still should be a follow-up evaluation to determine whether the behavior change has been incorporated into the client's lifestyle. This will determine the true value of the counseling.

Activity 5

PLANNING EFFECTIVE TEACHING STRATEGIES TO PROMOTE GOOD NUTRITION

EXAMPLE

As the visiting nurse in an agricultural area of the Pacific Northwest, you visit a Mexican-American migrant farm laborer, Jose H., his wife Rosa, and their three small children, ages five, four, and two. Rosa is five months pregnant. Their home base is Texas, but they move with the seasonal farm work. Their income is about $5000 per year. Both parents speak limited English, but have no reading skills in either Spanish or English. Mr. H. has been away from work for a week, which is why you were asked to call on them. Mr. H. is known to have had tuberculosis when he lived in Texas.

You note that your arrival is greeted politely, but distantly. Mrs. H. looks tired and pale. Mr. H. is lying in bed without moving at all. The room is very hot, and the children appear restless and irritable. Upon inquiry as to his illness, Mr. H. states that it is "empacho" and turns his head away from you. Mrs. H. says she thinks it is the bad air.

Step 1: Assessment

A. Sociocultural-economic factors: Mexican-American, Roman Catholic faith, migrant farm laborer, income below poverty level, five-person family, semi-illiterate. (Available from sources other than direct interviewing.)

1. What does this person want to learn, if anything? (He did not send for you; you were asked to check on him. At his point, he probably wants to learn nothing.)

2. Is he or is he not in crisis? (Observation would verify that he is. You now need to explore the meaning of "empacho" and "bad air.")

3. What is his definition of health and illness? (Interviewing skills are needed, but unless your culture is Spanish, his definition will vary considerably from yours.

4. What kind of communication does he respond to? (Adult, verbal skills in Spanish and English, no reading skills, pictures and other visual aids probably appropriate.)

5. What is his developmental stage? (Young adult.)

6. What gives meaning to his life? (Culture, social class, religion, environment, family structure.)

B. Medical history:

1. Past history of tuberculosis (from records).

2. For wife--four pregnancies in five years. May be a factor in later counseling, especially nutritional. Family planning is not a factor because of religious beliefs.

3. Immunization records for children; necessary information for later counseling.

4. Present illness--chief complaints.

5. Weight/height/digestion/elimination/appetite. You may need this information on other family members as well if counseling is done for entire family.

6. Hemoglobin and hematocrit would be helpful in the assessment.

C. Dietary history: Usually obtained by interviewing. Questions should elicit the following kinds of information:

1. Kinds of foods culturally acceptable; religious restrictions.

2. Meals: where eaten, when, with whom.

3. Food preparation--by whom, facilities for storage, safety.

4. Food budget--kinds of foods purchased; amount of money spent on food; other sources of food money, if any.

5. Typical day's meals: 24-hour recall, including snacks.

6. Food allergies, intolerances, dislikes.

Step 2: Planning

From the assessment summary, it becomes obvious that planning will need to take place around the family group, as the astute nurse will recognize that others besides Mr. H. have problems. The identified needs from this summary are:

1. Entire family has substandard diet. Diet history reveals diet lacking in several essential nutrients--namely, some amino acids, vitamins, and minerals (especially iron and calcium). Hemoglobin levels low for the mother and children. Cultural and socioeconomic factors have definitely affected their food habits.

2. Mr. H. has not stayed on his isoniazid therapy. Since he had been cured of tuberculosis, it was thought unnecessary. Culture affected this also, as he believes that once he has been treated, even by an x-ray for diagnosis, he has been cured.

3. Mr. H. has a gastrointestinal disease, probably an ulcer. Later diagnosis confirms this.

Note: At this point, the visiting nurse, if unfamilar with the culture, will need to do some research. "Empacho" refers to a gastrointestinal disease believed to be brought about by psychosocial forces such as eating food that is disliked, overeating, or from eating hot bread. Disease may also result from moving parts of the body from the normal position, or it may be caused by "bad air" entering a body opening.[4]

---

[4]Murray, R. and J. Zentner, *Nursing Concepts for Health Promotion* (Englewood Cliffs, N.J.: Prentice-Hall, Inc., 1975), pp. 292-293.

More research will also be necessary to obtain a list of foods that are culturally acceptable, are within financial means, and provide the deficient nutrients. A culturally desirable ulcer regimen will also need to be incorporated into the planning. Truly, all this is an imposing task, and some realistic compromises will have to be reached in order to succeed. The nurse may wish to seek the assistance of a dietitian at this point in the planning.

The behavioral objectives must be kept simple and realistic. The nurse will need to solicit cooperation and become a family friend before planning can proceed. The first objective might be a broad one, worked into with gradual shaping, with the others being added in small steps:

Objective:

Mrs. H. will be able to plan, prepare, and serve the family a balanced diet that is culturally desirable and within the financial limitations of the family.

Sub-objectives:

1. Can state what foods are needed to make the diet balanced nutritionally.

2. Can plan a day's menus using these foods.

3. Can demonstrate preparation practices that will conserve nutrients.

4. Can substitute foods of equal nutritional value that are acceptable to the family.

5. Can purchase or obtain foods that are needed to complete the family's requirements.

Each of these steps may take a lot of time, but there should be a reasonable time limit on each.

Objectives for the other listed problems can be added gradually. Mr. H.'s ulcer will heal without a special diet if his diet is balanced, although he may be more uncomfortable during the process.

Step 3: Implementation

Provided that good rapport was established during the planning stages, the nurse can next present Mrs. H. with the facts she needs to know by using posters, pictures, role playing, demonstrations, and the like and by providing opportunity for practice. A home health aide, preferably Mexican-American, can facilitate practice and furnish support and encouragement. Check other resources, such as the migrant council or Health, Education and Welfare services for additional aid to the family. The WIC (Women, Infants, and Children) Program could be of definite service. Usually a consulting dietitian is attached to this facility and can help the nurse with a lot of the implementation.

Step 4: Evaluation

Evaluation should be done after each step so that the teaching can be revised if the client has not understood. The evaluation should be documented in writing and passed to other members of the team along with a summary. Relevant feedback is a nursing responsibility. Follow-up visits by the visiting nurse and reports from other resource persons can validate whether learning has occurred. If the family diet improves and continues to be stable, if Mr. H.'s ulcer heals and he returns to work, and if subsequent visits show that the health of the family is good, then it can be assumed that the planned changes have been incorporated into the lifestyle of the family. The visiting nurse should remember that all change is slow and should try not to become impatient.

PROGRESS CHECK

From the following case study, devise a nutrition teaching plan using the four steps of the problem-solving process discussed in Activity 5.

> Debbie A. is a 16-year-old Caucasian from an upper-middle-class family. She is an only child, and both her parents are professional people who commute to their jobs from their pretentious home in the suburbs of a large midwestern city. She is in the tenth grade and makes good grades. She reports to you, the school nurse, on three consecutive mornings because she has an upset stomach and feels dizzy. She states that she "probably has the flu." Her temperature is normal. She reveals that she feels okay later in the day, but hasn't any appetite. You inquire about her menstrual period, and she finally admits that she has "missed twice." You suggest a free clinic for teenagers, which she visits, and a diagnosis of pregnancy is confirmed. She refuses to tell her parents, any of her friends, or her boy friend. She won't have an abortion and is ambivalent about keeping her baby or giving it up for adoption. In the meantime, you realize that she needs diet counseling very much, as she and the baby are at high risk. Her diet is typical of many teenage females in this culture, nutritionally inadequate and interspersed with periods of dieting. When you mention diet counseling to her, she gets very hostile and says she will continue dieting so that people will not find out about her condition.

ANSWER

Many satisfactory plans can be made for this case, but they should include the following information:

Assessment

Data needed:

1. Socioeconomic, cultural, religious, ethnic factors; environment, family structure; and so on.

2. Answers to the six questions related to the total person.

3. Medical history.

4. Dietary history.

Assessment summary:

Sixteen-year-old pregnant female, unwed, Caucasian from an upper-middle-class family. Only child. Parents well educated. Does not appear to have strong family ties and is alone much of the time. Communication with family poor. Religion not stated, assumed Protestant. Does not want an abortion. Is in emotional crisis. Medical history unremarkable. Is less than ideal weight for height and body build. Appetite poor. Diet history reveals poor knowledge of balanced nutrition, inadequate food consumption, and ignorance of the crucial function of food in pregnancy.

Planning

1. Spend time establishing rapport and confidence. Gain her participation in planning.

2. Research diet needed for pregnant adolescent if not known.

3. Look for other resources to give her support and financial assistance if parents do not help.

4. Set up behavioral objectives in writing. Plan content to help meet these objectives. Set time limits. There is need for immediate action here.

Implementation

Given Debbie's educational level, discussion and printed materials can be used in presentation, but a group approach might be more suitable. Recommend that she attend prenatal classes, preferably a class for girls in her age range. Group therapy can give powerful support and encouragement in her crisis.

Evaluation

Devise any suitable method to determine whether she has met the objectives. Follow-up will be a necessary part of her counseling, not only to evaluate learning, but also to provide her with a support system and increase her ability to cope with the situation.

Evaluate your effectiveness in being nonjudgmental and in communicating across your own cultural and social barriers.

POSTTEST

1. Compare and give one example of the differences between biological necessity and cultural patterning.

2. Explain the impact of culture on the development of eating habits.

3. Explain the significance of economics on food consumption.

4. Identify the factors that affect planned changes in eating habits.

5. The six questions relevant to the assessment of the total person are:

6. Name at least four useful items of information provided in a dietary history.

ANSWERS

1. Biologic necessity refers to the amount and kind of nutrients needed by the body to maintain life and health, while cultural patterning establishes values and beliefs about what is acceptable as food. Among numerous examples, a striking one is that of the Hindu who is suffering from protein-Calorie malnutrition, but will not eat meat even though many animals roam the countryside. Because they are considered sacred, the animals are well fed with grain that the Hindu should eat himself.

2. Acculturation is the way people are adapted to their environment and social order. It includes the way they are taught to regard what is acceptable as food and what is to be rejected, as well as all the religious and symbolic connotations attached to food.

3. Economics is especially significant in the food consumption of individuals and groups. It affects the kinds and quantities of food purchased, prepared, and served. It also affects the attitudes and adaptive mechanisms of a population or an individual within that population.

4. Awareness of personal and societal values, biological need, environment, cultural patterning, and governmental or industrial actions affect changes in food consumption.

5. (1) What does the person want to learn, if anything?

   (2) Is he or is he not in crisis?

   (3) What is his definition of health and illness?

   (4) What kind of communication does he respond to? (Education level, age, language, and so on.)

(5) What is his developmental stage?

(6) What gives meaning to his life? (His culture, social class, religion, environment, and the like.)

6. Kinds of food culturally acceptable.

Any religious restrictions.

Meals--where eaten, when, with whom.

Preparation--by whom, facilities for storage, methods, safety.

Amount of money spent for food, kinds of food purchased.

Typical intake--a 24-hour recall, including snacks.

Food allergies, dislikes, intolerances.

Handicaps that may interfere with eating (such as lack of teeth; paralysis of arm, hand, throat; and so on).

REFERENCES

Gifft, H., M. Washbon, and G. Harrison. *Nutrition, Behavior and Change*. Englewood Cliffs, N.J.: Prentice-Hall, Inc., 1972. Pages 115-122, 258.

Mason, M., et al. *The Dynamics of Clinical Dietetics*. New York: John Wiley & Sons, Inc., 1977.

Murray, R. and J. Zentner. *Nursing Concepts for Health Promotion*. Englewood Cliffs, N.J.: Prentice-Hall, Inc., 1975. Chapters 10, 11, and 12.

Robinson, C.H., et al. *Case Studies in Clinical Nutrition*. New York: Macmillan Publishing Co., 1977.

Robinson, C.H. and M.R. Lawler. *Normal and Therapeutic Nutrition*. 15th ed. New York: Macmillan Publishing Co., 1977. Pages 214-236.

Williams, S.R. *Nutrition and Diet Therapy*. St. Louis: The C.V. Mosby Co., 1977. Chapters 13 and 14.

SUGGESTED READINGS

Brink, Pamela, ed. *Transcultural Nursing: A Book of Readings*. Englewood Cliffs, N.J.: Prentice-Hall, Inc., 1976.

Redman, B.K. *The Process of Patient Teaching in Nursing*. St. Louis: The C.V. Mosby Co., 1976.

Overview of Therapeutic Nutrition

PEGGY STANFIELD, M.S., R.D.

CONTENTS

INTRODUCTION

Therapeutic nutrition is based on modifications of the nutrients in a normal diet to meet the individual's needs in a specific illness. The reader must comprehend normal nutrition and metabolism before the principles of diet therapy will be clear. She will also need to apply nursing knowledge of disease entities and related anatomy and physiology.

The purpose of diet therapy is to restore or maintain good nutritional status. It may be accomplished by modifying

1. One or more of the basic nutrients,
2. The energy value (Calories),
3. The texture or consistency, or
4. The seasonings.

In adapting the normal diet to deviations from health, any of the modifications, singly or in combination, may be needed to restore or maintain the good nutritional status of a given individual. In addition, therapeutic diets must be individualized, taking into account not only physical factors and the specific disease, but the patient's total acculturation as well.

The nurse's role is critical in helping a patient adjust to a modified diet. She is often the coordinator, interpreter, and teacher.

Meeting the patient's nutritional needs involves the coordination of the medical, dietary, and nursing staff. In the larger hospitals, the nurse maintains liaison between patient, physician, and dietitian; assists the patient at meals; observes the patient's response to meals; charts pertinent information; and supports and supplements the primary instructions given by the dietitian. In small hospitals, nursing homes, and community nursing services, the professional nurse may be responsible for the planning, supervising, and teaching of the modified diet. In many cases, she may need to interpret the diet into food selections, not only for the patient, but for the kitchen personnel as well.

The nurse, because of her constant and intimate association with a patient, can be the greatest factor in the patient's successful adjustment to his diet.

PREREQUISITES FOR THIS MODULE

The student should have completed a recent college-level course in normal nutrition and the module in this book entitled "Internal and External Factors Affecting Food Consumption."

TERMINAL OBJECTIVES

Upon the completion of this module, the learner will be able to:

1. Identify the principles of diet therapy.
2. Explain the purpose of diet therapy.
3. Describe the methods used to adapt a normal diet to the disease condition.
4. Recognize the most common therapeutic diets used in a clinical setting.
5. Formulate a plan to help a patient adjust to a therapeutic diet.

PRETEST

Before beginning this module, take the following pretest. If you are able to answer all of the questions correctly, you need not complete this module; go on to the next module. The correct answers follow the Pretest.

1. What is the major principle of therapeutic nutrition?

2. State the purpose of diet therapy.

3. Describe the methods used to adapt a normal diet to a disease condition.

4. The most common therapeutic diets are modified in what four ways?

5. Identify four illness factors that affect food consumption.

6. Explain the nurse's role in helping a patient adjust to a therapeutic diet modification.

ANSWERS

1. Therapeutic nutrition is based on modifications of the nutrients in a normal diet.

2. The purpose of diet therapy is to restore or maintain good nutritional status.

3. The diet should be altered to the specific disease (pathophysiology).

   The diet should be individualized to the patient's psychological, cultural, and socioeconomic conditions.

4. (1) Modified by altering basic nutrients.

   (2) Modified by altering energy value.

   (3) Modified by altering texture or consistency.

   (4) Modified by altering seasonings.

5. (1) Fear changes attitudes and personality.

(2) Immobilization compounds nutritional problems.

(3) Drug therapy may affect intake and utilization.

(4) The disease process modifies food acceptance.

6. The nurse has a key role. She assists the patient at mealtimes and explains, interprets, and supports both the physician's orders and the efforts of the dietary staff. She observes and charts pertinent information and coordinates the team. She involves the patient in his own care and provides a care plan for other staff members to follow. She plans for discharge teaching and follow-up.

ACTIVITY 1

PRINCIPLES AND PURPOSES OF DIET THERAPY

The care of the hospitalized patient takes into account physiological, psychological, and cultural factors as well as social and economic factors. Illness may alter any of these factors.

The stress of illness brings about many fears in the hospitalized patient and often causes personality changes. Immobilization brings about nutritional stresses that compound the original problem. In addition, drug therapy often affects food intake and interferes with nutrient utilization. The disease process itself modifies food acceptance. Food preferences may revert to those of earlier developmental stages. Symbolic security foods may be desired, or the fears that beset the patient may be expressed in terms of rejection and hostility regarding his food and resentment toward everyone connected with it.

Adding to these sometimes overwhelming stresses is the frequent necessity to modify the diet. When confronted with this necessity, patients frequently respond with inappropriate behavior and an unwillingness to accept the change. By recognizing the many factors that affect the hospitalized patient and helping him work through them, one can often help the patient accept his modifications more readily. In this milieu, the nurse becomes the key to the success or failure of the regimen.

The patient's nutritional needs must be identified from information regarding his past nutrition practices as well as his present illness. If his nutritional status was poor before admission, then his needs will be greater than those of the patient whose nutritional reserves are optimal. Individual analysis will be necessary.

The focus of diet therapy is on the patient's identified needs and problems. The diet ordered should be relevant to the nature of the illness and its effects on the body. It should be based on sound, scientific rationale in line with current nutrition concepts. It should not be the whim of the practitioner providing the care. The nurse has the right to question diets that are ordered for patients when there is no apparent link between them and the disease. Furthermore, the patient should be given an explanation of the reasons for his diet and the expected outcome from the change.

PROGRESS CHECK

1. List five factors that affect the nutritional care of the hospitalized patient.

2. How does the stress of illness affect food acceptance?

3. What is the focus of diet therapy?

4. Upon what principle is therapeutic nutrion based?

5. What is the purpose of diet therapy?

ANSWERS

1. (1) Cultural aspects.

   (2) Socioeconomic background.

(3) Psychological factors.

(4) Physiological makeup.

(5) The stress of illness.

2. (1) The patient is often fearful and rejects hospital food.

(2) Immobilization brings about nutritional stress.

(3) Disease process alters food acceptance.

(4) Medications may interfere with nutrient utilization.

3. Diet therapy focuses on thc patient's identified needs and problems.

4. Therapeutic nutrition is based upon modifications of the nutrients in a normal diet.

5. The purpose of diet therapy is to restore or maintain good nutritional status.

Activity 2

METHODS OF ADAPTING NORMAL DIETS TO DEVIATIONS FROM HEALTH

The basic concept in planning a therapeutic diet is that it is based on a normal balanced diet. The regular or house diets used in acute-care settings can be modified to meet specific conditions since they are already balanced diets. In addition to meeting specific needs, the changes that may be needed must take into account the total person.

Briefly, the modifications most generally used deal with four aspects:

1. *Modifying basic nutrients.*

The diet may need to be increased or decreased in protein, fats, carbohydrates, vitamins, or minerals. An increase would be needed to correct deficiencies or provide extra nutrients for repair of body tissue. The increase could be for a single nutrient, but more often it is for a combination, as the nutrients have interrelated functions. Examples include high-protein, high-carbohydrate, and high-vitamin diets following a surgery or diets high in iron containing foods when iron-deficiency anemia exists. If the patient is malnourished when admitted, the diet may require increases in all the nutrients. It would seem that increases in diet would be readily accepted by the patient, but this is not necessarily true. The patient with a chronic, debilitating illness may be anorexic and present quite a challenge to the staff. Nutrients are usually decreased to adjust the food intake to the body's ability to metabolize them. Examples include lowering the carbohydrate intake in a patient who has elevated blood sugar because the sugar cannot get into the cells or lowering fat intake because of elevated serum lipids. Renal diseases, which reduce the kidney's ability to excrete excess minerals may require a diet with lowered mineral content.

2. *Modifying energy value.*

When it becomes necessary to adjust the caloric content to bring about changes in body weight, the calculated diet is used. Calculations are based on the fuel factor of foods--the number of Calories per gram a food will furnish when metabolized by the body. Adjustments are made in the amounts of carbohydrate, protein, and fat contained in the diet. Examples include the underweight patient who may need a 3000-Calorie diet or the overweight patient who may need only 1000 Calories. The diabetic diet is also a calculated diet. The nutrient values are calculated individually in order to be sure that daily requirements for each are met. It is quite possible for a 1000-Calorie diet to be all fat and carbohydrate without significant protein foods if the nutrient content is not calculated for balance. Patients with certain malabsorptive disorders may require diets with increased energy value along with adjustments in the amount of a specific nutrient.

3. *Modifying texture or consistency.*

This modification is used to provide ease of chewing, swallowing, or digestion; to rest the whole body or an affected organ; or to progress a patient back to a regular diet. It is widely used in combination with other modifications. Examples include low-residue, soft, and liquid diets. Patients with gastrointestinal diseases as well as patients who have trauma to the mouth or throat frequently have the texture of their diet altered. Postsurgery patients may progress from liquid to soft to regular diets, as tolerated. Patients with cardiovascular disorders may require texture modifications to provide ease of digestion to rest the damaged heart.

4. *Modifying seasonings.*

Seasonings are usually adjusted to individual tolerances, but a few may be contraindicated in certain diseases. Salt restriction may be necessary for the patient who has decreased ability excrete it or who has edema or ascites, from whatever cause. Certain spices are thought to be contraindicated in gastrointestinal disorders such as ulcers and acute gastritis.

Whatever the modification, the goal of diet therapy remains the same: to restore and maintain good nutritional status. Whenever the diet imposes severe restrictions, the patient's appetite is poor, or absorption and metabolism are impaired, it is essential to recognize the need for dietary supplements such as vitamins, minerals, or high-protein concentrates.

A correctly planned diet is successful only when it is eaten. The diet must be individualized to take into account the psychological and cultural factors that influence food acceptance. In addition, the food must be attractive, palatable, and safe. The patient's environment at mealtime is also an important factor, as is the attitude of the persons who serve it.

PROGRESS CHECK

1. What are the basic modifications made in a diet?

2. Give an example and the rationale for decreasing a nutrient in the diet.

3. Name three situations where diet supplementation would be needed.

4. Explain how a diet can be individualized and still provide the correct modifications.

ANSWERS

1. Modify basic nutrients.

   Modify energy value.

   Modify texture.

   Modify seasonings.

2. There are numerous examples that would be correct. Your answer should satisfy you.

3. (1) When the diet imposes severe restrictions.

   (2) When the patient's appetite is poor.

   (3) When digestion, absorption, or metabolism are impaired.

4. Within the framework of the correctly modified diet, the individual's likes, dislikes, and tolerances should be built in. Foods of equal value should be substituted to meet his ethnic and cultural desires. Participation by the patient in choosing foods within the specified diet is desirable.

ACTIVITY 3

THE NURSE'S ROLE IN PATIENT ADJUSTMENT

The nurse, because of her position on the health-care team, can assist the patient in adjusting to his modified diet. She need not single out this need from other aspects of his care, but should remember to include it. The modified diet may be needed by the patient for weeks, months, or even a lifetime. He may need guidance in improving his normal diet. Whatever the need for diet instruction, it can be given as a adjunct to other teaching, with its importance properly emphasized.

Since learning about his needs begins with a patient's admission, it should follow through his hospital stay and include plans for discharge. Follow-up in the home environment may be necessary. The nurse in the acute-care setting should know how to plan for the patient's rehabilitation.

To ensure continuity of care from admission through discharge, a nursing-care plan is used. There are several acceptable kinds of plans, depending primarily on the institution. Generally, a plan will consider

1. Goals
2. Identified needs
3. Relevant background knowledge
4. Nursing activity
5. Approach
6. Results

Nutritional needs are a part of the total plan of care. For the purpose of this activity, we will emphasize only the nutrition aspect of the care plan in order to acquaint the student with the kinds of nutrition information that are pertinent.

Situation:

> Mrs. J., a 65-year-old widow, is admitted to your floor. She lives alone in a rented apartment. Social Security is her only income. She is overweight, hypertensive, short of breath, and has cataracts. She has been a diabetic for 15 years.

CARE PLAN FOR MRS. J. (EMPHASIS ON NUTRITION)

GOAL

1. To rehabilitate her to her highest potential (long range).

2. To restore and maintain good nutritional status.

NEEDS

1. Therapeutic nutrition
   a. To reach ideal weight
   b. To reduce sodium intake
   c. To control diabetes

RELEVANT BACKGROUND INFORMATION

1. A 2 g sodium, 1200-Cal. diabetic diet will fulfill these requirements. The diet prescription will require 125 g carbohydrate, 60 g protein, and 50 g fat. The P/S ratio for fat will be 1:1.

RELATED NURSING ACTIVITY

1. Diet history
2. Analysis of eating habits
3. Explanation of diet
   a. Reasons
   b. Expected outcome
4. Plan for diet instructions
5. Follow through on diet instructions
6. Discharge plan

APPROACH

1. Verbal exchange; Mrs. J. does not see well.
2. Positive approach. Find some good things she has been doing. Respect likes and dislikes.
3. Establish trust. Show concern. Work toward raising patient's self-esteem.
4. Clinical conference with dietitian.
5. Support, supplement instructions, facilitate feedback. Help patient to participate in selection of foods if menu available.

6. Include the diet follow-through and situational aids as needed.

RESULTS

Results depend on the patient's degree of acceptance and motivation to follow the diet. If an approach did not work, find another. Evaluation after instruction is necessary. Follow-up evaluation is also needed. Were the goals reached? Was good nutritional status restored? Will the patient maintain it after discharge from the hospital?

PROGRESS CHECK

Write a brief nutrition-care plan for the following patient:

Jack D. is admitted to the hospital through the emergency room, having received compound fractures of both legs in a motorcycle accident. He is 19, 6 feet tall, and weighs 140 lb. He has a past history of drug abuse, though at present he does not appear to be under the influence.

Care Plan for Jack D.

Goals

Needs

Relevant Background Information

Related Nursing Activity

Approach

Results

ANSWER

Your plan may vary with your own creative ideas, but in general it should address itself to the following information:

Goals

Same as example.

Needs

1. Therapeutic Nutrition

   a. To reach ideal weight

   b. To repair/replace cells

   c. To promote bone formation

   d. To restore nutritional reserves

Relevant Background Information

A diet modified by increasing the basic nutrients will be necessary. Based on his sex, age, height, weight, and the amount of trauma, plus the past history of drug abuse, the diet should contain approximately 3500 Calories, be high in protein (100-125 g), high in carbohydrates, and high in vitamins and minerals, especially iron, calcium, potassium, the B complex vitamins, and ascorbic acid. Interval nourishments are probably desirable.

Related Nursing Activity

Same as example.

Approach

Your choice.

Results

Your estimate.

POSTTEST

1. State the principle that should guide the planning of therapeutic nutrition.

2. State the purpose of diet therapy.

3. List two major factors that should be observed when planning modified diets.

4. List the four most common diet modifications.

5. List four ways in which illness alters a person's food acceptance.

6. List three terms that identify the key role the nurse plays in the patient's adjustment to diet modifications.

ANSWERS

1. Therapeutic nutrition is based on modifications of the nutrients in a normal diet.

2. The purpose of diet therapy is to restore or maintain good nutritional status.

3. (1) The diet should be altered to the specific disease (pathophysiology).

   (2) The diet should be individualized to the patient's psychological, cultural, and socioeconomic conditions.

4. (1) Modified by altering basic nutrients.

   (2) Modified by altering energy value.

   (3) Modified by altering texture or consistency.

   (4) Modified by altering seasonings.

5. (1) Fear changes attitudes and personality.

   (2) Immobilization compounds nutritional problems.

   (3) Drug therapy may affect intake and utilization.

   (4) Disease process modifies food acceptance.

6. (1) Coordinator

   (2) Interpreter

   (3) Teacher

REFERENCES

Robinson, C.H. *Normal and Therapeutic Nutrition.* New York: Macmillan Publishing Co., 1977. Chapter 27.

Williams, S.R. *Nutrition and Diet Therapy.* St. Louis: The C.V. Mosby Co., 1977. Chapter 23.

SUGGESTED READINGS

Murray, R., and J. Zentner. *Nursing Concepts for Health Promotion.* Englewood Cliffs, N.J.: Prentice-Hall, Inc., 1975. Chapter 5.

Redman, B.K. *The Process of Patient Teaching in Nursing.* St. Louis: The C.V. Mosby Co., 1976.

Weight Control

PEGGY STANFIELD, M.S., R.D.

CONTENTS

INTRODUCTION

In 330 B.C. Socrates said: "Beware of foods that tempt you to eat when not hungry and liquors that tempt you to drink when not thirsty." This may be the earliest recorded evidence of man's interest in controlling weight, which remains today a most popular subject to the layman and health professional alike. One might assume that in some 2300 years the problem would have been solved. Instead, as civilization progresses, the problem becomes greater and more complex.

This module is designed to give the nursing student some insight into today's problems involving weight control and some measures for therapeutic intervention in the client's behalf. Since approximately 60 million people are overweight and at one time or another a majority of the U.S. population are on weight reduction diets, it is important that nurses learn the principles of weight control.

The facts concerning weight control and longevity are significant in the nurse's education. Abundant statistical evidence indicates that obesity reduces life expectancy as well as the quality of life. Obesity increases the risk of a number of diseases, including diabetes, hypertension, atherosclerosis, gallbladder disease, renal disease, gout, and other degenerative diseases. Obesity complicates respiratory difficulties, such as emphysema, asthma, and chronic bronchitis. In the obese person who is free of respiratory disorder, the work of breathing is increased and lung volume is decreased. The hazards of surgery, pregnancy, and childbirth are multiplied by obesity. The psychological consequences of obesity can be devastating in terms of distortion of body image and negation of self-esteem. The obese often suffer discrimination in obtaining jobs, and their life insurance premiums are higher. Obesity is a very expensive phenomenon --mentally, emotionally, physically, and financially.

Obesity exists for a number of reasons, but one significant factor is the body's need for fuel. Foods provide the energy that fuels the human machine. The human machine is turned on at conception and runs continually until death. The body must have a constant fuel source, or else it will die;

being a highly efficient machine, it provides itself with fuel storage--the adipose tissue cells. Unlimited quantities of reserve fuel to meet future energy needs may be stored in these cells. The amount stored depends on the amount taken in and not needed at the time of ingestion.

Weight control remains a prime concern of health professionals everywhere, as well as of the public at large. Methods for controlling weight have proliferated over the years, as evidenced by the innumerable diet regimens that exist in the American culture. In spite of the more than $20 billion spent each year by consumers for diet pills, exercisers, special equipment, books about diets, magic potions, and miracle weight-loss regimens, the success rate for the control of obesity is very poor. In fact, the problem of obesity looms in ever increasing proportions.

Other forms of treatment have included diets, drugs, hormones, starvation, surgery, psychotherapy, self-help groups, and exercise programs. Most of these have low success rates. The three methods most commonly used by health professionals at this time are (1) managing eating behaviors (behavior modification) with adjunct psychotherapy, if needed; (2) reducing total caloric intake while maintaining a balance of essential nutrients (the clinical approach); and (3) specific, individually designed metabolic approaches. These three approaches will be discussed in greater detail in the activities that follow.

PREREQUISITES FOR THIS MODULE

Successful completion of a recent college-level course in normal nutrition will be necessary. In addition, an approved nutrition textbook and the American Dietetic Association's Exchange Lists for Meal Planning are helpful resources. The 1976 revised edition will be most helpful, although older editions may be used. These lists may be obtained from either of the following organizations:

The American Dietetic Association
430 N. Michigan Ave.
Chicago, IL 60611
(Fifty cents per copy)

American Diabetes Association, Inc.
1 West 48th Street
New York, NY 10020

TERMINAL OBJECTIVES

Upon the completion of this module, the learner will be able to:

1. Explain the importance of weight control throughout the life cycle.

2. Describe the role of energy metabolism in weight control.

3. Identify clinical, metabolic, and behavioral methods of controlling weight.

   a. Calculate food allowance for a reduction diet using a standard exchange list.

   b. Use simple behavioral techniques to provide psychological support.

4. Apply scientific principles to diet regimens in order to assess their value.

5. Provide diet counseling to clients, and successfully use the techniques of weight control for oneself.

PRETEST

Before beginning this module, take the following pretest. If you are able to answer ten out of the twelve questions correctly, you need not complete this module. The correct answers are given following the Pretest.

1. List and briefly explain two reasons why weight control is important throughout the life cycle.

2. Identify two factors that may lead to developmental obesity.

3. Three social and cultural factors that contribute to patterns of obesity are:

4. List (a) three psychological factors crucial in the development of obesity and (b) three psychological factors that thwart subsequent control of obesity.

5. List three metabolic factors believed to be implicated in the development of obesity.

6. Briefly explain the laws of energy that affect weight control

7. Compare the clinical, metabolic, and behavioral methods of controlling weight.

8. List the data needed to provide a basis for calculating a reduction diet.

9. Upon what basis is the food allowance for reduction diets calculated?

10. Calculate the energy value of 100 g of carbohydrate, 60 g of protein, and 50 g of fat.

11. Explain the behavioral approach to controlling obesity.

12. Describe (a) two scientific principles useful in evaluating the merits of reduction diets and (b) three characteristics that would be indicators of fraudulent claims for reduction diets.

ANSWERS

1. Statistical evidence indicates that obesity (1) shortens the life span and (2) reduces the quality of life. More specifically: (1) obesity complicates diseases and increases the risk of their development; and (2) obesity is devastating from a psychological standpoint, and it is financially debilitating.

2. (1) Overfeeding in infancy.

   (2) Establishing abnormal eating patterns in early childhood.

3. (1) Type of diet ingested: Americans have high fat diets and snack patterns with caloric density.

   (2) Patterns of exercise: most sports are the spectator type; activity for physical fitness is sporadic and is not emphasized for the population most needing it.

   (3) Motivation: obesity is more socially acceptable among lower socioeconomic groups; weight control is undertaken for the wrong reasons in the upper classes.

4. a) (1) Boredom

      (2) Loneliness

      (3) Anxiety

      (4) Also, frustration, sorrow, avoidance, discontent, etc.

   b) (1) Feelings of hopelessness regarding success in losing weight.

      (2) Feelings of conflict about being controlled by other people.

      (3) Extremes of mood.

5. (1) The obese person's inability to convert foods to heat production.

   (2) Alterations in blood lipids that favor increased formation of fatty tissue.

   (3) Overloading metabolic pathways for carbohydrates and fat so that lipogenesis is favored.

6. Energy is neither created nor destroyed, but it may be constantly transformed. If energy is not used, it will be stored. There will always be a balance. Any program that cannot account for energy balance will not work.

7. The metabolic method of controlling weight is designed to take into account those metabolic factors believed to be involved in excess weight gain. The diet includes a fasting period to break the metabolic pattern of lipogenesis, a six-meal plan to reduce overloading, and a supplement of polyunsaturated fats to accelerate the oxidation of body fat. This differs from the clinical approach, which is based upon energy exchange and the client's situational needs. The clinical method uses the standard exchange system and is calculated by prescription. Except for the amount of total Calories, both the metabolic and the clinical diets meet the standards for balance set up by the Food and Nutrition Council. The behavioral method varies from the other two by approaching weight control with techniques designed to change eating behaviors that are maladaptive. It may be used successfully in combination with either the metabolic or the clinical approach.

8. The first thing needed is an extensive diet history, which should reveal how much the person has actually been eating. Next, we need information about the person's activity. Third, a measurement of the basal metabolic rate should be taken. This may be an exact laboratory measurement or an approximate assessment. Data about the person's situational, cultural, and

economic status will be helpful in planning and in facilitating the subject's cooperation. Most of this information can be acquired with the diet history.

9. The food allowance for reduction diets is calculated from the nutritional and caloric values from the American Dietetic Association's exchange system and the recommended daily food guide.

10. 1090 Calories

$$\begin{aligned} 100 \times 4 &= 400 \\ 60 \times 4 &= 240 \\ 50 \times 9 &= \underline{450} \\ & \quad 1090 \end{aligned}$$

11. The behavioral approach to control of obesity is based on learning psychology. It involves an educational approach to self-management, as well as a change in lifestyle. Basic, simple techniques for changing maladaptive eating patterns are given to the client after these behaviors have been identified. The client must make a commitment to accomplish certain goals, and these goals are put into a written contract.

12. a) The scientific principles listed may include any of those principles that relate to the energy laws--balance, conservation, transformation, and so on--as well as those that relate to the properties of foods--their composition and functions in the body. Also helpful is a knowledge of the physiology of the body.

    b) The characteristics of fraudulent books are numerous, but three major ones are:

        (1) Unproven and unsubstantiated claims for a food, product, pill, or other as yet unrecognized therapeutic agent.

(2) Endorsement or coauthorship by an authority figure with either real or bogus credentials.

(3) Abundant testimonials and/or successful cases on record.

ACTIVITY 1

REGULATING FOOD INTAKE THROUGHOUT THE LIFESPAN

The best treatment for obesity is prevention, and so the most vigorous efforts to prevent obesity should be directed toward the most susceptible groups. The most critical periods for development of obesity are (1) during childhood, especially infancy and early puberty; (2) for the female, especially after the first birth and after menopause, due to hormonal changes; (3) for the male, the period between ages 25 and 40, due to decreased activity and unreduced caloric intake. Both sexes tend to gain after age 50, due to a lowered basal metabolic rate and decreased activity.

Developmental Obesity

The pattern of obesity is often set in infancy because of the parents' erroneous belief that a fat baby is a healthy baby. Abnormal eating patterns may also be established because the mother assumes that any sign of distress means that the baby is hungry. Recent evidence indicates that the number of fat cells may be determined early in life. Metabolic feeding studies in young children suggest that the number of fat cells can be increased by overfeeding and decreased by underfeeding. This number of cells remains constant throughout adulthood, so overfeeding in infancy may lead to obesity in adulthood.[1] Obesity of this type is sometimes referred

---

[1]Young, E.A., et al., "The endless fight against fat," *Current Prescribing*, March 1976, pp. 49-50.

to as *constitutional obesity* but more often as *developmental obesity*. By either name, it constitutes a barrier to weight reduction. The young obese person may reduce the size of the adipose cells, but still have a large mass of them. The ratio of body fat to lean body mass may also be greater than in the lean child, so that body composition must be considered when attempting weight reduction. The percentage of obese children who remain obese into adulthood is significantly greater than the percentage of lean children who become obese as adults.[2]

Cultural and Social Factors

Cultural and social conditioning can contribute to the problem of obesity. Social and cultural factors affect the type of diet ingested, the patterns of exercise, and the motivation of individuals to control their weight. These factors must be taken into account when planning treatment.

In the American culture, sedentary occupations, effortless transportation, spectator sports, television, radio, and movies all contribute to the incidence of obesity. In addition, the American diet is high in fat, which contributes to caloric density and makes many extra calories easy to consume. Physical fitness has been emphasized for American youth in recent years, but attention has not been focused on the obese child who needs it the most.

Obesity is more prevalent among the lower socioeconomic groups, and this tendency is more pronounced among women than men. It also appears that obesity is more socially acceptable and less rigidly discouraged among lower social classes.[3] In the higher-income groups, greater social value is placed on being slim.

Psychological Factors

Psychological factors are crucial in the development of obesity and its subsequent control. The

---

[2]Young, p. 50

[3]Gifft, H., et al., *Nutrition, Behavior and Change* (Englewood Cliffs, N.J.: Prentice-Hall, 1972), p. 159.

nurse must be aware of these factors at all times in order to maintain therapeutic interventions. The individual who is bored, lonely, feeling unloved, discontented, anxious, frustrated, experiencing sorrow, or avoiding the realities of life may turn to eating as a solace. Psychological factors thwarting the control of obesity include a feeling of hopelessnes regarding success in losing and maintaining the loss, a feeling of conflict about being controlled by other people, and the obese person's tendency toward extremes of mood. These mood swings are usually reflected in the way individuals diet, such as eating nothing all day and then consuming huge amounts of food in the evening.

In addition, disturbances may occur after weight reduction. Concern over changed body image, especially in the juvenile, may be manifested as anxiety, distrust, or aggression. Preoccupation with food can be carried to extremes, especially in the young female, resulting in anorexia nervosa. This psychosomatic disorder, once believed rare, is now being diagnosed with increasing frequency.

Finally, some obese patients have an unconscious fear of losing weight. They may have many conflicts regarding personal relationships, especially those of a sexual nature, and as long as they remain encased in adipose tissue, they will not be expected to confront or resolve them.

Inheritance Factors

While it is generally agreed that environmental factors contribute to at least 98 percent of all cases of obesity, genetic influences provide an interesting and less explored part of the total picture. It is difficult to prove that genetic factors alone can account for obesity. The nurse, however, should be aware of the more significant of these genetic factors in order to deal more effectively with the problem.

Several investigations have found a high correlation between obesity in parents and obesity in their children. This could be due to the effects of excessive food preparation and consumption. However, this propensity for obesity was not seen in adopted children in these families, and the opposite was found to be true of identical twins reared apart. These studies strongly suggest there is a genetic factor in obesity.[4]

Metabolic Factors

Reduced thermogenesis--a situation where less food energy is converted to heat and more is stored as body fat--has been cited as a metabolic factor in obesity. After normal persons eat a meal, there is a 25 to 50 percent increase in body heat production. In obese individuals, this increase is much less marked.[5] Another explanation offered is that the metabolic pathways for carbohydrate and fat become overloaded so that lipogenesis is favored. Some obese patients have shown alterations in blood lipids that suggest the increased formation of fatty tissue.[6] Finally, a feeding pattern marked by decreased frequency and consumption of a large nutrient load at any one time is shown to be associated with increased lipogenesis.

PROGRESS CHECK

1. List three critical periods for the development of obesity during the lifespan and cite one reason for each period.

---

[4]Young, pp. 49-50.

[5]Young, pp. 49-50.

[6]Robinson, C.H., *Normal and Therapeutic Nutrition* (New York: Macmillan, 1977), p. 408.

2. ___ Developmental obesity is believed to

   1) Increase the number of fat cells.
   2) Increase the size of the fat cells, but not the number.
   3) Decrease the lean body mass, as fat replaces lean.
   4) Lead to obesity in adulthood.

   Choose the correct answer from among the following:

   a) 1 and 3
   b) 2 and 4
   c) 1 and 4
   d) 2 and 3

3. Identify three factors in the American culture that contribute to the incidence of obesity.

4. ___ Obesity is more prevalent among

   1) Lower socioeconomic groups.
   2) Men.
   3) Women.
   4) Children.
   5) The wealthy.

   Choose the correct answer from among the following:

   a) 1 and 3
   b) 2, 3, and 5
   c) 1 and 4
   d) 3 and 5

5. ___ Psychological factors that are detrimental to controlling obesity include

   1) Feelings of conflict.
   2) Mood swings.
   3) Feelings of hopelessness
   4) Low self-esteem.

Choose the correct answer from among the following:

a) 1 and 3
b) 2 and 4
c) 1, 2, 3, and 4
d) 4 only

6. ______ True or False?

The behaviors that follow weight reduction are very positive changes, especially among the young.

7. ______ True or False?

There is no evidence to indicate that obesity may be inherited.

8. ___ Metabolic factors that may contribute to the incidence of obesity include:

1) Excessive food consumption.
2) Inability of the body to absorb foods efficiently.
3) Inability of the body to convert food energy to heat.
4) Excessive rate of formation of lipids.

Choose the correct answer from among the following:

a) 1 and 3
b) 2 and 4
c) 1 and 2
d) 3 and 4

ANSWERS

1. (1) Infancy and early puberty--overfeeding of infants and children; crisis periods of adolescence.

   (2) Female, after first pregnancy and post-menopausal--hormonal changes.

(3) Male, ages 25 to 40--decreased activity, same caloric intake.

(4) Both sexes after age 50--lowered BMR, decreased activity.

2. c

3. Any of the following: sedentary occupations, effortless transportation, spectator sports, television, radio, movies, high fat intake, lack of exercise.

4. a

5. c

6. False

7. False

8. d

Activity 2

PHYSICAL FACTORS IN WEIGHT CONTROL

The treatment of obesity is based on the laws of energy. Energy is neither created nor destroyed, but is constantly transformed. Since it is never lost, it must either be used or stored. The energy equation will always balance. Any weight control program that cannot account for energy balance will not work.

For the purposes of this activity, we will agree on the following:

1. The caloric values of nutrients are calculated at 4 Cal/g for carbohydrate and protein and 9 Cal/g for fats (1 Cal = 1000 cal or 1 kcal). Though not considered a

nutrient, alcohol will account for approximately 7 Cal/g, and it must be considered when calculating caloric intake.

2. Energy expenditure for an individual is based on his basal metabolic rate plus an allowance for activity.

3. A key number in weight control is 3500, the number of Calories of energy in a pound of body fat.

Caloric values for foods have been standardized over the years. While there may be some variance in the total caloric value of a given foodstuff, it is usually slight.

The basal metabolic rate (BMR) for an individual may be accurately assessed under the ideal conditions of a laboratory setting. There are, however, many approximate methods, and they encompass a broad range of averages. Deutch provides a simple rule for calculating the BMR.[7]

For women: Add a zero to your weight in pounds. To the result, add your weight in pounds.

Example: For a 135 lb woman, add a zero, which gives 1350. To this, add 135 to get a BMR of 1485 Calories.

For men: Add a zero to your weight in pounds. To the result, add twice your weight in pounds.

Example: For a 150 lb man, add a zero, which gives 1500. To this, add 300 to get a BMR of 1800 Calories.

To correct the BMR for age, reduce it by 2% for every decade past 20 years of age.

---

[7]Deutch, Ronald M., *Realities of Nutrition* (Palo Alto: Bull Publishing Co., 1977), p. 65.

Example: If the BMR is 1800 Calories at age 20, at age 30 it would be 98% of 1800 or 1764 Calories.

Added to the caloric expenditure for the BMR is the expenditure of Calories for activity. While most of us would like to think that we engage in moderate to heavy activity, the fact is that a low level of activity is the usual pattern. Thus, the normal level of activity is considered by the Food and Nutrition Council to be "very light."[8] This basic activity rate averages approximately 30 percent of the BMR per day. If we use this shortcut method and go on with our examples from above, the woman would add 445 Calories to her BMR for activity and the man would add 540 Calories. It is obvious that if we intend to effect a caloric deficit, increased activity is an important step.

A pound of body weight equals 3500 Calories. The basis for this is calculated as follows:

1 lb fat = 454 g

1 g fat = 9 Cal

However, body fat contains some water and is therefore calculated at 7.7 Cal/g.

454 g x 7.7 Cal = 3496 Cal/lb body fat

A 500-Calorie deficit per day amounts to a 3500-Calorie deficit per week, which produces a loss of one pound of body weight per week. This would result in a weight loss of 52 pounds per year.

In order to lose two pounds of body weight per week, 1000 fewer Calories than the amount expended would need to be ingested daily. Then 52 pounds of body weight could be lost in six months. Of course, this drastically curtails the food intake. Some people prefer to set intake at only 500 Calories below BMR expenditure and to work out an exercise program to use up the other 500 Calories per day. If the exercise program is maintained, the result will be the same.

---

[8]Deutch, p. 65.

In order to see how easily weight is gained, let us look at the opposite kind of calculation. The consumption of two extra 10-oz glasses of a regular carbonated beverage per day would add approximately 250 extra Calories per day to the diet. This would amount to an excess of 3500 Calories in two weeks or the gain of one pound of body weight every two weeks. This would equal a weight gain of 26 pounds a year. In approximately four years, there would be a 100-pound wieght gain.

To carry this idea one step further, let us look at the common myth that proposes that everyone gets "middle-age spread." While it is true that the BMR slows with age and caloric intake must be lowered accordingly, consider the following calculation. A 20-year-old person with an ideal weight who gains only two pounds a year until the age of 45 will be 50 pounds overweight going into the middle years. It is therefore obvious that, if the energy laws are ignored, obesity can begin at any age.

PROGRESS CHECK

1. ___ The ingestion, absorption, and metabolism of a hamburger on a bun with mustard which contains 30 g of carbohydrate, 14 g of protein, and 10 g of fat will yield

   a) 175 Calories.
   b) 266 Calories.
   c) 321 Calories.
   d) 500 Calories.

2. ______ True or False?

   A 20-Calorie mint candy and a 20-Calorie serving of carrots contain the same amount of fuel value.

3. Using the shortcut method outlined in this activity, perform the following computations:

   a) Figure your BMR energy needs according to your sex, age, and weight.

b) Add the caloric expenditure for your activity to your BMR. Figure this at the basic or "very light" activity rate. If you feel that the rate for very light activity is too low for you, you may use any chart that gives Calorie expenditure per minute for vigorous activities. Remember that the only time you can count is the time you are actually performing the activity, not the resting times in between. For example, it is estimated that when amateur players engage in an hour of tennis, each player spends about six minutes in actual vigorous activity.

4. ___ Mary's caloric intake for a 24-hour period is 2400 Calories. Her caloric expenditure during this same time is 2150 Calories. If this daily pattern continues at the same rate, how long will it take Mary to gain five pounds?

a) 26 days
b) 10 weeks
c) 26 weeks
d) 1 year

<u>ANSWERS</u>

1. b	30 g CHO	x	4 Cal/g	=	120 Cal
	14 g PRO	x	4 Cal/g	=	56 Cal
	10 g FAT	x	9 Cal/g	=	90 Cal
					266 Cal

2. True

3. a) Add a zero at the end of your weight in pounds. If female, add your weight to this result. If male, add double your weight to this result. Reduce the total by 2 percent for every decade past 20.

   b) Figure 30 percent of your BMR and add it to the BMR figure. This will approximate your total energy expenditure per day. If you choose to add more vigorous activities, total the amount of time spent actually performing these. Multiply by the number of Calories used per minute and add to the above total.

4. b 250 Calories per day in excess of needs equals 3500 excess Calories (or one pound of fat stored) every two weeks. It would therefore take ten weeks to gain five pounds.

Activity 3
WEIGHT-REDUCTION REGIMENS

The Metabolic Diet

The nurse who chooses to work in an institution where a metabolic clinic is utilized is more likely to encounter a metabolic type of diet, although it may be used in any hospital with medically selected and supervised patients. The diet will depend upon the clinician and the type of patient.

One such diet is the Gordon diet[9] used at the University of Wisconsin Medical School. It includes an initial 48-hour fast to break the metabolic pattern of lipogenesis; a pattern of six daily meals (of equal size) to reduce glucose overloading; salt

---

[9]Williams, S.R., *Nutrition and Diet Therapy* (St. Louis: The C.V. Mosby Co., 1977).

reduction (2-3 g); and a high-protein, moderate-fat, low-carbohydrate food intake. This diet includes a supplement of polyunsaturated fatty acids to accelerate the oxidation of body fat. Total caloric intake is 1320 Calories per day.

The diet meets or exceeds the Basic Four standards for balance and, with the exception of Calories, will meet the recommended daily allowances prescribed by the National Research Council. It is, however, not situationally adaptable and usually cannot be fitted into the client's individual desires or cultural patterns. In may be economically infeasible, as it requires eleven ounces (cooked weight) of lean meat daily plus egg, fruit, and vegetables for nutritional balance and seven teaspoons of unsaturated fats. The client would need a high degree of motivation and constant reinforcement and supervision for the diet to be successful.

Clinical Method: The Exchange System

The most common approach to the control of obesity is based upon energy exchange (Activity 2) and the client's situational needs. It is referred to as the clinical approach.

The exchange system was set up by the American Dietetic Association and other professional organizations. It is the accepted system for all calculated diets, including diets for diabetes. The exchanges are based on simple groupings of common foods having generally equivalent values. Each group's values are expressed in terms of grams of carbohydrate, protein, and fat as well as in Calories. Foods may be exchanged only within the same group. There may be some variations between the values given in the exchanges and those given in the appendices of textbooks; for simplicity in calculation, however, standard values are used.

The 1976 exchange revision included some changes designed to bring about closer agreement with current nutritional knowledge. The main changes occurred in the milk and meat categories along with a total reorganization of the vegetables to eliminate the A and B groupings. Values for the six food groups, according to the 1976 revision, are as follows:

FOOD	APPROXIMATE MEASURE	CHO (g)	PRO (g)	FAT (g)	CALORIES
1. Fruit Exchange	Varies	10	-	-	40
2. Bread Exchange	Varies	15	2	-	70
3. Meat Exchange					
Lean	1 oz	-	7	3	55
Medium Fat	1 oz	-	7	5	75
High Fat	1 oz	-	7	8	100
4. Milk Exchange					
Nonfat	1 cup	12	8	-	80
Low Fat	1 cup	12	8	5	125
Whole Milk	1 cup	12	8	10	170
5. Fat Exchange	1 tsp	-	-	5	45
6. Vegetable Exchange	½ cup	5	2	-	25

Certain raw vegetables for salads and other items containing negligible carbohydrate, protein, and fat are listed in "free" groups. You may refer to these when planning menus.

When the exchange method is used, the calculation of a diet requires that the nurse refer to the nutritional values of the foods. Diets are dictated somewhat by client preference, but in general they should follow the daily food guide for the type of food and the amount to be included. The exchange list differs from the daily food guide in one aspect: the milk group in the daily food guide includes cheddar and cottage cheese, but these are listed with protein foods in the food exchange lists.

The following is a sample calculation for a 1200-Calorie reduction diet.

The prescription for this 1200-Calorie diet is 125 g carbohydrate, 60 g protein, and 50 g fat.

Carbohydrate

125 g x 4 Cal/g = 500 Cal

Protein

60 g x 4 Cal/g = 240 Cal

Fat

50 g x 9 Cal/g = 450 Cal

1190 Cal per day

	FOOD	EXCHANGES	CHO (g)	PRO (g)	FAT (g)
CARBOHYDRATE Prescribed total = 125 g	Milk (skim)	2	24	16	-
	Fruit	3	30	-	-
	Veg.	2	10	4	-
			64		
CHO from milk, fruit, veg. exchanges = 64 g 125 - 64 = 61 61 g CHO to be supplied by bread exchanges Amount of CHO in 1 bread exchange = 15 g $\frac{61}{15}$ = 4 bread exchanges	Bread	4	60	8	-
			124		
				28	
PROTEIN Prescribed total = 60 g PRO from milk, veg., bread exchanges = 28 g					

	FOOD	EXCHANGES	CHO (g)	PRO (g)	FAT (g)
PROTEIN (Continued) 60 - 28 = 32 32 g PRO to be supplied by meat exchanges Amount of PRO in 1 meat exchange = 7 g $\frac{32}{7}$ = 5 meat exchanges	Meat (med. fat)	5	-	35 63	25 25
FAT Prescribed total = 50 g Fat from meat exchange = 25 g 50 - 25 = 25 25 g FAT to be supplied by fat exchanges Amount of FAT in 1 fat exchange = 5 g $\frac{25}{5}$ = 5 fat exchanges	Fat	5	-	-	25 50
	Total g		124	63	50

Total Calories

Carbohydrate

124 g x 4 Cal/g = 496 Cal

Protein

63 g x 4 Cal/g = 252 Cal

Fat

50 g x 9 Cal/g = 450 Cal

1198 Cal per day

The exchange list for the day obtained from these calculations is then translated into food terms. The following is an example:

BREAKFAST	LUNCH	DINNER
½ c milk, skim	1 c milk, skim	½ c milk, skim
½ c orange juice	1 small apple	½ banana
½ c oatmeal	½ c carrots	½ c green beans
1 boiled egg	1 slice bread	½ c mashed potatoes
1 slice bacon	2 oz tuna fish	1 dinner roll
2 tbs cream	2 tsp mayonnaise	2 oz roast beef
Coffee	Dill pickles	1 tsp butter
	Iced tea	Diet soda

TOTALS

2 milk (skim) exchanges
3 fruit exchanges
2 vegetable exchanges
4 bread exchanges
5 meat exchanges
5 fat exchanges
Free items

The total exchanges for the day should be checked against the calculations. Unless this check is made, it is easy for beginning practitioners to add two or three extra exchanges, which would exceed the desired caloric intake.

The Behavioral Approach to Obesity

Although behavior modification is not new in learning theories, only in recent years has its usefulness in treating obesity been recognized. It is primarily a treatment modality based on social learning theory. One of its main principles is that any behavior regularly repeated is most likely to be rewarding in some way. Because eating behavior is learned, maladjustive eating behavior can be unlearned. Behavior modification involves an educational approach to self-management coupled with a change in lifestyle. It can be used with almost any client because the principles are simple and basic.

It can also be used by groups and, once the principles are identified, may be used by the client alone. Weight loss is self-reinforcing.

The first step in using behavior therapy is to determine the behaviors that contribute to overeating and lack of exercise. Lists are kept by the client that record these behaviors as well as the feelings that bring about the eating behaviors. These observations become the baseline for the future plan.

Second, the client, with the therapist facilitating, chooses the target behavior. This is defined specifically: how much weight loss over what period of time? The established goals must be realistic and within reach. There should be short-term objectives as well as a long-term goal. Each time an objective is attained, a reward significant to the client is provided. The reward may differ with each client.

Third, the therapist discusses with the client simple behavioral techniques that can be used to manage the problem behaviors. A major technique is called "cue elimination." Many things have become cues to start eating, such as TV watching, seeing food, buying and preparing food, and so on. Methods for eliminating these cues include avoiding contact with the situations or avoiding foods that stimulate eating. Other techniques may include slowing the pace of eating, leaving some food on the plate, eating in only one place in the house, storing food in opaque containers, not shopping when hungry, and a host of other techniques as needed by the individual for special situations.

Finally, a written behavioral management contract is drawn up. This is a commitment on the part of the client to fulfill the goals agreed upon by the client and the therapist. It includes the reinforcers (rewards) for desirable behavior as well as the consequences for undesirable behavior. The plan is reviewed at regular intervals by the therapist and the client, and the plan is negotiable.

The following case study shows the use of behavior modification principles and includes some client reeducation concerning balanced nutrition.

Dianne S. is 37, an R.N. with two boys ages 10 and 12. She was divorced three months ago. She works full time at a mental health clinic. She has a heavy case load and works long hours. She also takes calls on weekends. While she is home, she bakes for the boys for the coming week, usually cookies, breads, cakes, and the like. She is taking a graduate class one night a week at a nearby university. Dianne has gained 20 pounds in the past four months. She realizes that the increase in weight has come about because of a drastic change in her life-style, and she decides to replace her recently acquired habits with more appropriate ones. She wants to shed the 20 pounds, buy a new wardrobe, and develop some new social interests. She comes to you for behavior therapy.

Step 1

You advise her to keep lists to establish a baseline. A week later she returns her chart to you. The table on page 176 is a compilation of the seven days, which were all fairly much alike.

Step 2

The target behaviors are chosen.

Long-term goal: Twenty-pound weight loss in 10 weeks.

Short-term goal: Two-pound weight loss per week.

Rewards: Short-term--a new article of clothing, under $15, for each two-pound weight loss.

Long-term--at the end of ten weeks, if the 20-pound weight loss is attained, assess present wardrobe and complete it with new clothes. Make travel arrangements for a trip.

Consequences for not reaching goal--no new clothing for that week nor at the end, plus no trip.

TIME OF DAY	MINUTES SPENT EATING	ACTIVITY WHILE EATING	LOCATION WHILE EATING	FOOD TYPE, QUANTITY	EATING WITH WHOM	FEELING WHILE EATING	EXERCISE TYPE, AMOUNT
7:00 a.m.	5	Standing	Kitchen	2 c coffee with cream	Alone	Hurried	
9:00 a.m.	10	Talking on phone	Office	2 doughnuts 1 c coffee with cream	Alone	Anxious	
1:30 p.m.	10	Driving	Car	3 cookies 1 apple 1 bag peanuts	Alone	Depressed	
5:30 p.m.	15	Studying	Kitchen	2 rolls 2 pats butter Tuna noodle casserole 1 c milk	Boys	Frustrated	
10:00 p.m.	30	Watching TV	Living room	6 oz wine 8 crackers Cheese spread 1 pc cake Few nuts 1 pc choc. candy	Alone	Lonely, bored	

Step 3

The behavioral techniques are chosen:

1. Eat in only one place in house--kitchen chosen.

2. Lunch may be eaten in the car, but a different type of lunch must be carried from home. Eat slowly. Stop car when eating. Suggestions for more appropriate foods are given at this time:

   Protein foods such as cheese, eggs
   Raw vegetables such as celery, carrots,
     cauliflower
   Fruits, apple okay
   Thermos with skim milk

3. Arise 30 minutes early. Prepare breakfast (suggestions for appropriate breakfast foods given). Sit down to eat with boys. Eat slowly. Talk to boys.

4. Omit midmorning snack. A larger breakfast should make this easier to accomplish.

5. Add one daily exercise: a bicycle ride with children of not less than one mile after work each day except school night.

6. Increase length of evening meal from 15 to 30 minutes. Eat slowly. Savor food. Visit with boys instead of studying. Avoid distractions while eating. Add vegetables to evening menu. Limit food items to one serving of each per meal (no extra roll, butter, and so on).

7. Avoid late evening snacks. Indulge in activity other than eating while watching TV. Chosen: knitting new sweater for herself.

8. Change type of food prepared on weekends while on call. Chosen: freeze-ahead casseroles--protein items and vegetables. Change children's snack patterns to fruit, nuts, and the like to promote better nutrition for them.

9. Change shopping behaviors. Avoid buying soda pop, candy, chips, chip dip, spreads, and other nutrient-deficient foods.

10. Plan activities to socialize more.

11. Identify feelings that bring about inappropriate eating behaviors and substitute a more suitable activity. Keep a list of satisfactory experiences that can be used again.

12. Keep a log, diary, or other accurate record of food eaten and activities performed.

13. Keep a weekly weight chart posted in a prominent place (bathroom or kitchen).

Step 4

Draw up the written behavioral contract. Include:

a. Weight-management goals (long- and short-term)

   (1) Observed caloric intake
   (2) Increased physical activities
   (3) Eating-habit changes

b. Rewards

   (1) Short-term (weekly) reward is $15 clothing item
   (2) Long-term (end of ten weeks) reward is

      (a) Complete new wardrobe
      (b) Take a trip

c. Consequences for not reaching goal

   (1) No shopping for clothes
   (2) Cancel travel plans

d. Review of progress dates

e. Renegotiation, if agreed to by both parties

f. Signatures

In providing diet counseling for clients, you will find the following management techniques for controlling obesity helpful:

1. Provide a specific diet, acceptable to client.

    a. Balanced nutrition
    b. Adaptable to his environment
    c. Culturally desirable
    d. Economically feasible

   An extensive dietary history will give you much of this information. You will need considerable knowledge of food values.

2. Employ behavior therapy.

    a. Open relationship with client
    b. Techniques for behavior modification
    c. Periodic reviews of progress

3. Recommend daily exercise, according to individual's tolerance. You may need to make a careful physical assessment before recommending certain types of exercise.

4. Provide support and encouragement. Assess significant others in the client's environment who can also supply these essentials and enlist their aid. A partner is a boost to the commitment to lose weight.

5. After significant weight loss has occurred, if the client still has inner conflicts and appears insecure, unhappy, and fearful, the therapist can safely assume that inner changes have not kept pace with outer changes in behavior. Psychotherapy may be recommended at this point, either in private sessions or at a community mental health center.

It is obvious that both the clinical and the behavioral approach to the control of obesity will require a lengthy program. This is the advantage they enjoy over other forms of weight control. An extended program gives the client time to permanently change his habits, and a better chance of remaining in control. The expected outcome is better health through balanced nutrition and balanced weight.

PROGRESS CHECK

1. ___ The purpose of dividing the metabolic diet into a six-meal pattern is to
   a) Prevent hunger.
   b) Reduce glucose overloading.
   c) Break the pattern of lipogenesis.
   d) Balance the diet.

2. ___ The inclusion of a supplement of polyunsaturated fatty acids in the metabolic diet is believed to
   a) Accelerate the oxidation of body fat.
   b) Reduce glucose overloading.
   c) Break the pattern of lipogenesis.
   d) Balance the diet.

Questions 3 through 8 relate to the following situation:

> Marvin C., a 57-year-old truck driver, is admitted to the hospital for diagnostic studies. He is 5 ft, 10 in tall and weighs 220 pounds. The doctor orders a diet for weight reduction. The prescription is 150 g carbohydrate, 70 g protein, and 70 g fat. Marvin admits to you that he has been on reduction diets before but can't stay on them.

3. ___ The caloric value of the diet is
   a) 1000 Cal.
   b) 1200 Cal.
   c) 1500 Cal.
   d) 1800 Cal.

4. Using the sample calculations given in this activity as a guide, set up the diet in terms of food exchanges to meet his diet prescription.

a. Number of milk exchanges ____.

Type of milk ____________.

b. Number of fruit exchanges ____.

c. Number of vegetable exchanges ____.

d. Number of bread exchanges ____.

e. Number of meat exchanges ____.

Type of meat ______________.

f. Number of fat exchanges ____.

5. ___ Since Marvin says he has been unable to stay on a reduction diet in the past, you decide to incorporate some behavior modification into the teaching you will do before he goes home. In order to gain his cooperation, you will describe behavior modification as

a) A treatment.
b) A disciplinary measure.
c) A reeducation project.
d) A psychiatric therapy.

6. ___ Marvin wants to try behavior modification as part of his therapy. Before you can counsel him, you will need to know which of the following?

   1) How much weight he should lose.
   2) His eating habits.
   3) His eating patterns
   4) His feelings regarding eating and weight.
   5) What kinds of activities and objects are significant to him.

   Choose the correct answer from among the following:

   a) 1, 2, and 4
   b) 3 and 5
   c) 1 only
   d) All five

7. A major technique used in behavior modification is the elimination of cues that stimulate eating. Which of these will you use for Marvin?

8. List five things to be included in the written behavioral contract.

ANSWERS

1. b

2. a

3. c

4.

	CHO	PRO	FAT
a. 2 milk exchanges, low fat (2%)	24	16	10
b. 3 fruit exchanges	30		
c. 1 vegetable exchange (see note below)	5	2	
d. 6 bread exchanges	90	12	
e. 6 meat exchanges, medium fat		42	30
f. 6 fat exchanges			30
	149	72	70

Total caloric intake = 1514 Cal/day

5. c

6. d

7. Your decision must be individualized to the cues that you recognize when Marvin gives you the information to establish his baseline.

8. Weight-management goals, long- and short-term:

   (1) Rewards

   (2) Consequences

(3) Review dates

(4) Renogotiation agreements

(5) Signatures

Activity 4

THE PROLIFERATION OF FAD DIETS

This activity should bring into focus for the student the realities of dieting and the myths, fallacies, and fads that permeate American culture. The realities are much harder to live with than the myths. Many people deal in wishful thinking, attaching themselves to exaggerated claims for any concoction, drug, food combination, or chemical reaction that promises quick weight control results without any conscious effort on their part.

The harsh realities of dieting are succinctly phrased by Fineberg: "The patient must be made to understand that if he is to reduce his weight, keep it down and not harm himself in the process, he must practice the self-discipline that is needed to adhere to a balanced diet of reduced caloric content."[10] Implied in this statement are the determination, motivation, and willpower needed to change one's lifestyle and eating habits forever.

If people truly believe that weight control is essential to their health, then why do the myths persist? The answer, while not satisfactory, is probably that sooner or later the person concludes that the treatment is worse than his fear of the consequences. Having reached that conclusion, he still has nagging doubts, and thus he is a prime candidate for all the literature that promises an easy way out.

A second major reason for the failure to successfully control weight may be that nutrition is a

---

[10]Fineberg, S.K., "The realities of obesity and fad diets," *Nutrition Today*, July/August 1972. Reprinted in Labuga, T.P., *The Nutrition Crisis, A Reader*, p. 296.

relatively new science. Knowledge in the field of nutrition is still hazy and incomplete; there are gray areas. There are phenomena for which the cause is unknown. The results of the current intensive scientific research, which at a later time may become scientific truths, at present remain unproven. Most of the popular publications about obesity are based on unproven and unsubstantiated claims and scientific half-truths. Perhaps half of what they say is true, but the reader does not know which half. If you, as an informed student of health sciences, sometimes have difficulty separating fact from fiction, imagine the confusion that exists for the layman.

A third major reason for the failure of sensible, sound weight-control practices is the behavior of physicians. In recent years, the most criticized crash diet books have been written by doctors, and many of them have the word doctor in the title--*Dr. Atkins Diet Revolution, The Doctor's Quick Weight Loss Diet*, and so on. It is much easier to cope with fad diets written by quacks than with those sponsored or authored by an M.D. Most members of the medical community abhor this practice and are very verbal in their criticisms. However, their concern has not been translated into action. Medical schools do not require a course in nutrition, although the first White House Conference on Food and Nutrition in 1969 pointedly requested this curriculum change. In general, the physician's knowledge of nutrition is very fragmentary. Most of what he knows is highly theoretical, and he is unable to translate this theory into practical advice.

While the medical profession has had more than its share of overzealous and misinformed authors, it would be unfair not to mention that the nutrition profession produced one of the most prominent authors of nutrition and health books, who was considered by health authorities to be a food faddist and a charlatan: Adelle Davis. The space limitations of this activity preclude reviewing her books. Suffice it to say that these books are not recommended for the bookshelves of the professional health worker, the physician, or the public. If the student has read any of her publications and found them plausible, consider again the dilemma of the layman.

Some characteristics the student can look for in evaluating faddist publications have been described by Blackburn[11] and can be summed up as follows:

1. Involvement of a product or idea as yet unrecognized as being an effective therapeutic agent.

2. A semblance of authority: a bogus degree or other credentials or a recognized degree in a professional discipline irrelevant to the field in which the book is written; endorsement by an authority figure.

3. The citation of research and practices from institutions of renown (for example, the Mayo Clinic diet).

4. Development of seemingly plausible scientific mechanisms.

5. Provision for self-diagnosis and self-treatment; the making of cure-all promises.

6. Fostering of controversy with unqualified theses.

7. Undocumented claims of success through testimonial-type evidence.

8. Recommendations of dosages and products.

9. Appeal to the mass market: simple language; collaboration with a popular-style writer; jacket design for popular, not scholarly, appeal.

10. Claims for enhancement of sexual potency.

11. Prominent missionary zeal.

While not every publication may contain all of these characteristics, the appearance of three or

---

[11]Blackburn, H.W., *New England Journal of Medicine*, 283: 214, 1970. Reprinted in *Medical Opinion*, December 1972, p. 14.

more should cause suspicion, if not outright rejection, in the informed student. Perhaps the single most significant factor to guide the choice of a reduction diet is that it must lead to a lifetime change in eating habits and that this change must restore the individual to optimum potential. It is truly rehabilitation.

PROGRESS CHECK

The following excerpt is from an advertisement for a new book which sells for $9.95. Evaluate it using the criteria proposed by Blackburn and the scientific principles of energy metabolism.

> <u>WHAT MAKES SOME PEOPLE FAT, OTHERS SKINNY?</u>
>
> Have you ever wondered why some people put on weight almost no matter what they eat--while other people remain skinny while eating almost anything? Modern research shows that probably the most important factor in staying slim is your "metabolism"--that is, how well you "burn up" the foods you eat.
>
> <u>THE AMAZING DISCOVERY OF "NEGATIVE ENERGIZER FOODS"</u>
>
> Modern science has discovered that some foods actually help "spark" the fires of your metabolism to burn up the calories of other foods you eat.
>
> These foods are called "negative energizer" foods because they actually help your body burn up more calories than they themselves contain. Thus, the more you eat of these amazing, but common foods, the more weight you lose.
>
> <u>EAT WHATEVER YOU WANT</u>
>
> Absolutely NOTHING is forbidden on this diet. If you simply can't resist foods that tend to be fattening, you're shown how to mix them with the negative energizer foods to neutralize their fattening effects.
>
> Furthermore, in this new book, you'll discover . . .

A complete list of negative energizer foods you can obtain easily at your supermarket and produce stand.

How these negative energizer foods work to burn up more calories than they, themselves, contain.

How negative energizer foods should be mixed with your meals to enable you to lose two pounds a day --14 pounds a week--until you reach the weight you desire.

How negative energizer foods should be used to keep you slim PERMANENTLY.

Why you can enjoy as many as six meals a day--and as many snacks as you wish--as long as you mix in negative energizer foods.

How negative energizer foods can bring you added joy and pleasure in love and sex (see page 158 for an eye opening discussion of how nutrition and diet can affect your love life).

A special variation of the Negative Energizer Food Plan for those who want to lose a lot of weight (50 to 100 pounds or more).

TRUE CASE HISTORIES--DOCUMENTED AND ON FILE IN THE AUTHOR'S OFFICE FILES

Lillian P. was 50 pounds overweight. She suffered severe arthritis, high blood pressure, and other ailments that kept her constantly sick. Within three weeks of using negative energizer foods with her meals, she lost 30 pounds, and her distressing symptoms began to disappear.

Thelma R. was unhappy with her life and had eaten her way to over 220 pounds. She could not stop eating candy, cakes, and cookies between meals. Her husband had grown revolted by her and might even have begun seeing another woman. When she heard that she could eat as much as she wanted with the negative energizer food system, she was delighted and her fear of weight loss vanished. It took her only a few weeks to lose 80 pounds and once again regain her former weight of

140. Afterwards, her husband's romantic interest in her was rekindled more strongly than ever--and now he only has eyes for her

<u>A MEDICAL DOCTOR ENDORSES THIS EFFECTIVE "NEGATIVE" ENERGIZER" WEIGHT LOSS SYSTEM</u>

"[The author] seems to have captured in this book some of the latest scientific methods for not only controlling the body's weight, but for keeping it in good health, with a maximum amount of energy and well-being."

--W. Spencer Gurnee, M.D., F.A.C.S.

ANSWER

Remarkably, this synopsis of the book contains all eleven of the undesirable characteristics. In addition, it violates the scientific principles of balanced nutrition and flies in the face of the laws of energy metabolism. Finally, the term "negative energizer" is an attempt to put new life into old fallacies. The principle of the specific dynamic action of foods has been misconstrued in practically every faddist reduction regimen ever printed.

POSTTEST

1. a. Name at least three diseases that may develop or be complicated because of obesity.

   b. Give two examples of psychological disturbances that occur in the obese.

   c. List two ways in which obesity causes financial problems.

2. Describe three ways in which American sociocultural factors contribute to obesity.

3. Explain how the feeling of being unloved could be crucial in the development of obesity.

4. Three methods of controlling weight are in general use by health practitioners. Name them and give the rationale for each.

5. In order to make an intelligent choice of a reduction diet for a client, what data should the nurse have?

6. Suggest a more appropriate behavior modification for each of these statements made by a client:

   a. "I just can't get up in time to eat breakfast."

b. "I usually grab a bite of lunch on the run."

c. "I do the grocery shopping on my way home from work."

d. "Just thinking about my problem is so frustrating it sends me right to the refrigerator."

7. Develop a brief teaching plan for a client, focusing on adequate nutrition, but reducing caloric intake to bring about weight loss.

ANSWERS

1. a. Choose any three of the following: diabetes, hypertension, gallbladder disease, atherosclerosis, renal disease, respiratory disease, surgery, childbirth, gout, arthritis.

   b. (1) Distorted body image

      (2) Negative self-esteem

   c. Choose two of the following: increased medical bills, job discrimination, higher life insurance premiums, higher costs for larger clothes, higher food bills.

2. (1) Americans are very sedentary in their work and play. Technology has reduced the need for caloric expenditures.

   (2) The American diet is concentrated in calories, and unwise food choices are made either because of ignorance of food values or for convenience.

   (3) People in lower income brackets must stretch food dollars, so they buy less meats, vegetables, and fruits and more starches, sweets, fats, and "filling" foods. Also, it is more socially acceptable to be obese in this group. Higher income groups eat "status" and gourmet foods, which tend to be high in fat and calories.

3. A person who feels unloved feels unworthy, rejected, and isolated. These feelings lead to anger and self-deprecation. Eating is a solace, sometimes the only pleasure for such persons. If nobody cares what happens to them, neither do they. Becoming obese is a coping mechanism. It forms a facade to protect them from the fears associated with being hurt or rejected by another, failing in a job, or being sexually inadequate. Eating becomes the major comfort against all of life's problems.

4. Method / Rationale

	Method	Rationale
(1)	Metabolic	To provide the client with a diet regimen which will compensate for the metabolic disequilibrium believed to be a causative factor in obesity for some individuals.
(2)	Clinical	To provide the client with a calculated diet regimen which is based on thermodynamics and designed specifically for that individual.
(3)	Behavioral	To provide the client with some appropriate behavior modifications to eliminate or suppress maladaptive eating behaviors.

5. (1) Diet history

(2) Usual activity pattern

(3) Basal metabolic rate (exact or approximate)

(4) Cultural, social, and financial data related to the client

(5) Physical factors--height, weight, health status, and so on

(6) Amount of weight to be lost; diet prescription

(7) Criteria for evaluating various reduction regimens

6. a. Plan ahead to allow time for breakfast.

(1) Screen activities of the evening and decide which can be omitted to allow getting to bed earlier.

(2) Change schedule to arise a half-hour earlier.

(3) Prepare breakfast the night before.

b. Prioritize work time. Schedule lunch break. Avoid distractions. Eat leisurely. Emphasize time for self.

c. Avoid this behavior. Shopping when hungry results in overbuying and in buying inappropriate foods.

d. Find an activity, preferably physical, that will be substituted for eating when frustrated.

Other techniques that you may think of can be substituted for any of the above answers, as long as you feel that they eliminate or suppress the cues that bring about inappropriate responses.

7. Your plan might include:

	Action	Rationale
(1)	Provide a specific diet acceptable to client	To provide balanced nutrition adaptable to his environment, culturally desirable, and economically feasible.
(2)	Employ behavior therapy	To provide techniques for self-management of his diet and periodic reviews of his progress.
(3)	Recommend daily exercise to individual tolerance	To provide a safe way to burn up excess calories.
(4)	Assess significant others in client's environment.	To provide support and encouragement.

Action	Rationale
(5) Assess client behaviors after significant weight loss has occurred	To provide the therapist with evaluation of her teaching effectiveness. or To provide the client with opportunity for psychotherapy if needed.

REFERENCES

American Dietetic Association. *Exchange Lists for Meal Planning*. Rev. ed. Chicago: American Dietetic Association, 1976.

Deutsch, Ronald M. *Realities of Nutrition*. Palo Alto: Bull Publishing Co., 1976. Chapters 3 and 4.

Ferguson, J.M. *Habits, Not Diets, The Real Way to Weight Control*. Palo Alto: Bull Publishing Co., 1976.

Gifft, H., et al. *Nutrition, Behavior and Change*. Englewood Cliffs, N.J.: Prentice Hall, 1972.

Jeffrey, D.B., and R.C. Katz. *Take It Off and Keep It Off: A Behavioral Program for Weight Loss and Healthy Living*. Englewood Cliffs, N.J.: Prentice-Hall, 1977.

Labuga, T.P. *The Nutrition Crisis: A Reader*. St. Paul: West Publishing Co., 1975. Chapters 30, 31, and 32.

Robinson, C.H. *Normal and Therapeutic Nutrition*. New York: Macmillan, 1977. Chapter 29.

Shore, F.S., and J. Wischi. "Diet books: Facts, fads, and frauds." *Medical Opinion*, December 1972, p. 14.

Williams, S.R. *Nutrition and Diet Therapy.* St. Louis: The C.V. Mosby Co., 1977. Chapter 24.

Young, E.A., et al. "The endless fight against fat." *Current Prescribing*, March 1976, pp. 49-50.

SUGGESTED READINGS

Deutsch, Ronald M. *The New Nuts Among the Berries.* Palo Alto: Bull Publishing Co., 1977.

Lazarus, A. *Behavior Therapy and Beyond.* New York: McGraw-Hill, 1971.

Levitz, L.S. "Behavior therapy in teaching obesity." *Journal of the American Dietetic Association*, 62: 22 (January 1973).

Orr, Richard. "Anorexia nervosa." *Nursing Care*, October 1976, p. 28.

Shafer, R., and E. Yetley. "Social psychology of food faddism." *Journal of the American Dietetic Association*, 66: 129 (February 1975).

Stunkard, A.J. *The Pain of Obesity.* Palo Alto: Bull Publishing Co., 1976.